Harnessing Hope in Managing Chronic Illness

IØØ42521

Harnessing hope is fundamental to adapting to a chronic illness or palliative illness, and this fascinating book provides a new framework that will enable physiotherapists and other healthcare professionals to engage with patients to create better interactions and outcomes for rehabilitation.

Based on extensive research into how patients express their experiences, it identifies those factors that influence how hope can be used to benefit an interaction. It also considers central questions to illustrate how interactions can be psychologically mapped to assess emotions, adjustment, and hope. The book then features practical guidance on how to integrate the idea of hope into therapeutic conversations with patients, fostering acceptance and adaptation to the present, and looking towards the future.

This book will interest any practitioner working with patients experiencing chronic pain or palliative illness, as well as students across physiotherapy, occupational therapy, and community nursing. It may also interest any general readers facing challenges around trauma or loss.

Dr Andrew Soundy received his PhD from the University of Exeter, UK, in 2006. His interest in mental health during this time was ignited by a passion around the experiences of individuals with schizophrenia. He undertook his post-doctoral research at the University of Birmingham in 2005, with a focus on health psychology and physical activity. He began research on the concept of hope in 2009. His research has focused on chronic and palliative illness populations, often with a focus on neurological conditions. This work considers the experiences and perspectives of patients, caregivers, and healthcare professionals. The work has often been qualitative in nature, theory generating, and from 2019 onwards very applied to the pragmatic interactions of healthcare professionals. One of his greatest ambitions is to help healthcare professionals create more hopeful interactions with patients. To date, he has published over 120 articles and has experience working with global research groups and global organisations such as the World Health Organisation. His current research is devoted to improving patient interactions and training universities and NHS Trusts across the UK. This current book can summarise some of this focus and bring together essential developments from scholars studying the concept of hope and interactions from across the globe.

Harnessing Hope in Managing Chronic Illness
A Guide to Therapeutic Rehabilitation

Andrew Soundy

R Routledge
Taylor & Francis Group

LONDON AND NEW YORK

First published 2025
by Routledge
4 Park Square, Milton Park, Abingdon, Oxon OX14 4RN

and by Routledge
605 Third Avenue, New York, NY 10158

Routledge is an imprint of the Taylor & Francis Group, an informa business

© 2025 Andrew Soundy

British Library Cataloguing-in-Publication Data
A catalogue record for this book is available from the British Library

ISBN: 978-1-032-73826-0 (hbk)
ISBN: 978-1-032-73828-4 (pbk)
ISBN: 978-1-003-46616-1 (ebk)

DOI: 10.4324/9781003466161

Typeset in Times New Roman
by Apex CoVantage, LLC

During the most difficult and uncertain times in my life, I have found a firm foundation from my faith in Jesus. This book is dedicated to Him.

Contents

Preface

A lot of my past research has focused on chronic illnesses and the idea of hope and the ability to look forward. This research area is currently flourishing, but I felt the breath of understanding about this area was not yet fully utilised in practice to support people during times of suffering. During times of distress and suffering, the ability to look forward may seem impossible. Whilst someone may, in the right conditions, be motivated and energised to look forward, suffering in life, including experiences of illness, grief, loss of relationships, roles, or jobs, can place a big challenge on anyone wanting a similar view. Such moments may be complicated by additional stresses and challenges; people at such a time may lack energy; they may feel captive to their situation rather than being hopeful for the future, a hope for survival or a hope for the suffering to end may be more possible and may be all that can be seen. Another hope may appear for a quick fix or an end to the situation that has caused suffering. However, if the change does not come and nothing seems hopeful, an individual can feel and embody an experience of being completely broken and overwhelmed, without any perception of control or energy. This may be because of the different circumstances that have come at once or the depth and impact of a particular circumstance. At such a time, what may be possible is the ability not to give up, and that may take all the energy and effort that an individual has. Further to this, such situations may not pass quickly, and they may last for years. However, I believe that all people can change and that it is possible, even in such circumstances, to regain motivation and energy. That is not to say such experiences are forgotten; situations and circumstances we live through can become scars from the past, or like a mental pit or trap that can be fallen into. From my own experience, such instances reduce across time and can become less intensive or effective in stopping you, but the mental trap may not easily be forgotten.

I believe in the potential for people to change, and I believe that as a part of supporting people to access that potential, healthcare professionals need to have the communication tools which help them understand the challenges faced by people quickly and in a meaninful way. An important goal of the work is to reduce suffering and help people find meaning and motivation. The work has been developed to harness hope by focusing on a simple psychological assessment through listening and asking specific questions, which provide a map of how the individual is adapting to a challenge they are facing. What makes this work unique is how it draws on specific hope literature to understand and support challenges and difficulties faced by people with chronic illness. This book was written as a way to consider and develop hope-centred interactions. The work is aimed at generating meaningful interactions that consider if a difficulty or challenge requires further understanding. The work also highlights the importance of, and provides a way to capture essential concepts relating to psycholgoical and emotional adaptation as well as hope in relation to a named difficulty.

The main tool described in later chapters is named the model of emotions, adaptation, and hope (MEAH). The book provides some practical application of using the concepts in specific ways to aid conversations rather than providing a critical overview of the concepts. The term model may be misleading for readers in terms of comparing the work to other models of therapies. I wouldn't describe this work as therapy but as something to enhance understanding of how individuals are managing. The work is aimed at helping understand the process of adaptation and being able to support hope-centred interactions. The goal of many therapies is to change thoughts and behaviour, and they are often underlined by principles or conditions and often require a process of learning before application. Rather than focusing on where or how a patient needs to change, this work looks to help develop a need to focus on adaptation, hope and energy, and feelings to develop a good understanding around how an individual is responding to a challenge and then, if needed, further explore the situation for factors which may influence that and the possibility of creating goals. This process is short and enables meaningful conversations to be developed where an individual feels heard. The application of the work will help increase hope and trust in the practitioner as well as empower the individual to consider their future.

The psycho-therapeutic benefit for patients that has been identified when applying this work results from being heard and understood. The benefit for praciticioners has been reported as feeling more able to navigate difficult interactions. The development of the work has been within physiotherapy education, and the work has demonstrated that there can be an efficient, pragmatic way of identifying people who are in circumstances, which make feeling motivated and ready to progress with therapy very difficult or impossible. One of the guiding principles of the work is that a tool is developed that is easy to learn and can be applied in a single session. My research has shown that this can be learned quickly (<50 minutes of e-training) and delivered during a single short interaction. As part of the training now provided to physiotherapists across the UK, the work is used in different ways, including as (a) a screening tool (< 30 seconds), (b) a very brief therapy tool (applied in 10 minutes), or (c) an extended therapy tool where the understanding is considered in more depth and a goal is developed (applied in 30 minutes). The purpose of the main tool that is presented is to help start an interaction, create trust, and establish a relationship, where hope can flourish. The purpose of the extended version is to use a fuller understanding of hope and the factors that influence hope to help guide a meaningful conversation towards an identified goal. Where a goal is not identified, benefit has still been found. Finally, it is important to note that whilst the book is focused on chronic illness, the main model developed certainly has a broader application to consider how hope can be created and how psychological and emotional adaptation is understood.

CONTENTS

v

Contents

TABLES

PREFACE

THIS work had its origin in the concern of one of the authors about those children who entered a certain grammar school in a high position on the entrance list and who therefore gave promise of good academic progress, yet were found at the end of the first academic year to have a very low standard of attainment. This failure was coupled in the minds of these children with frustration, for a very high percentage of them left school at the earliest age permissible. Just at this time, government reports and large sociological surveys in England and Wales were much concerned with early leaving; and here, in a grammar school, was flesh for the bones of such reports and surveys.

Some of what is written in this work concerns the entrance examination to the grammar school, and this might appear to make the book irrelevant in these times of bilateral, multi-lateral and comprehensive tendencies. However, our main concern is with the forces which make or mar educational promise at that critical stage of a young person's life—the transitional stage from primary to secondary education. We have sought to discover the important influences and have tried to make some assessment of their relative strength. These influences are at work in all types of schools; some are in the material environment, some are in the personalities that surround us, some are born with us and some are acquired in the journey of life.

In our efforts to discover the main causes of educational deterioration (and as a by-product to the work, the causes of improvement) we had to get very close to the people concerned. We studied them in their school activities and went to see them in their leisure moments at home. We think that we came to know them. This procedure confined our work to a relatively small number of pupils; but we chose this method of study in depth rather than a more superficial treatment of a larger number. Both methods have their faults, and a combination of the two is usually desirable. Our resources were, however, quite inadequate for a large-scale survey and we made a virtue out of necessity. We also endeavoured to supplement the case-study technique by tests of statistical significance wherever these were appropriate.

We tender grateful thanks for co-operation to the County Medical Officer for information on health gradings; to the headmaster at the grammar school for class lists and tests; to the headteachers of junior schools for 'further information' on some of their pupils; and to parents for their helpful co-operation. For the typing of the manuscript and for some very efficient secretarial assistance at a late stage in the work we are heavily indebted to Mrs. R. M. Lewis. We thank Dr. Phillip Williams for kindly reading the typescript and making a number of useful suggestions. R. R. Dale also tenders his sincere thanks to the Department of Education and Science for making secretarial assistance available, and to the authorities of the University College of Swansea for putting extra accommodation at his disposal.

R. R. DALE
S. GRIFFITH

I

THE SCHOOL AND THE PROBLEM

Introduction

THIS book derives its inspiration from another which one of
its authors wrote some years ago.[1] The examination of the
transition from school to university which is described there
was meant, however, to be a broad survey of the whole problem
from both the research and educational points of view, with
here and there a much deeper analysis of special areas. Its
importance—if it be conceded that it had any importance at
all—was that it sought to integrate a whole group of related
problems, ranging from the teaching in the Sixth Form,
through the problems of selection and transition, to university
guidance and teaching and the final degree.

The present book again examines a transition, that from
primary to grammar school, but it makes no attempt to cover
such a wide range of problems, nor does it make detailed
analysis of previous research. It attempts rather to secure
additional evidence about the reasons for the success or failure
of pupils in the grammar school. In some cases the enquiry
leads back to the primary school, in others to an examination
of academic factors within the grammar school, in others to
the homes of the children. Always in the centre of the picture
is the child; John who is failing in spite of intellectual promise;
Mary who is succeeding in spite of her parents; David, dull
and industrious; Elaine, bright and lazy. In the centre is the
child, but on each side of him is a parent, and in the background
Society.

Many parents are deeply concerned about the educational

[1] Dale, R. R. *From School to University*, Routledge, 1954.

I

progress of their children, and this concern is probably greatest
about the time of the transition from primary to secondary
education. Though many of the problems of this period are
produced by the change from one school to another, their
satisfactory solution often depends, strangely enough, on the
home even more than on the school. They are problems in
which, wittingly or unwittingly, every parent plays a part. We
hope that those parents who read this book will become even
more discerning about the nature of the influence which they
exert, day by day and in thousands of little ways, on the
educational progress of their children. For although the school
provides the machinery, the mainspring comes from the home.
Behind the failure of a child often lies the failure of a home;
conversely the success of the child often springs from the support
given by understanding and loving parents. Although 'we
cannot alter where we will', and a parent may be in the clutch
of circumstances beyond his control, yet many a parent may
be helped by reading why others have failed and others have
succeeded. This world is so made that there is little in human
affairs that is certain; parents may try hard and fail abysmally
through no fault of their own, but if the way to success is
charted the chances of safe arrival are increased.

Parents are as varied as the human race. Some are intel-
lectuals and some are not; some are educationalists and some
would refute the description with decided vigour, but nearly
all are interested in their children. This interest will lead some
of them to read this book. In doing so those whose vocations
are in a different walk of life may find here and there passages
which are too technical because they are written for more
specialised readers. They are encouraged to omit these and turn
to those sections of the book which describe the problems as they
existed in the lives of the parents and children. Though the
care which the authors have taken to preserve the anonymity
of the participants has deprived the book of some of the colour
and drama of real life, this was a price which could not be
avoided. Much remains, however, to give human significance
to the statistics.

For specialised readers who have not read the brief note in
the preface on the limitations of this study we would emphasise
that we have been concerned with one grammar school only.

In this school we have examined the total entry for five consecutive years, discovered 39 'deteriorators' as later defined, and have explored in detail the factors associated with their deterioration. At the time the study was commenced this approach was somewhat new. At a later stage we added, for contrast, case studies of 10 'improvers' and certain information about 26 additional 'improvers'. When these numbers became sub-divided into various categories they were inevitably small. We are well aware of the dangers connected with the use of such small numbers. We therefore present our results as the story of what we found within our five-year population. Where figures for sub-groups are excessively small we acknowledge that a freak of chance or a misjudgment in classification might well double the figures in another five-year sample or in another school. These however are for the less important sub-groups, and the figures for the main groups are sufficiently large to enable us to present findings for our sample which are reliable and which we hope will be of interest to parents, educationalists, sociologists and social workers.

Purpose of the Survey

We have seen that the investigation was begun as a case study of the reasons for the marked deterioration of certain pupils who entered the grammar school in a fairly high position on the entrance list. It was observed that only a few of those who deteriorated in the first year at the school recovered academically during subsequent years at the school; also, there seemed to be a tendency for them to leave the school at the first opportunity. Out of eleven such academic deteriorators who entered the school in Year 1, eight had left by the end of the academic Year 4, and one more left during Year 5, before his G.C.E. examination. Out of seven entries of Year 2 who subsequently deteriorated academically, four had left by the end of Year 5, and two left during the next school year before their G.C.E. examination.

Deterioration Defined

The deteriorators were arbitrarily and objectively defined for

3

all five years of the study according to a demotion criterion. This criterion needs a little explanation.

Demotion and promotion in the grammar school were begun in the first term as a result of the end of term examinations; further demotion and promotion took place at the end of the academic year. These processes were therefore accelerated in this grammar school, as compared with most others, where the first reconsideration of the streaming occurs at the end of the first year. This accelerated procedure proved to be helpful to the enquiry. In Years 1, 2, 3 and 4 there was a three-form entry, and 'deteriorators' were defined as pupils who had been demoted by the end of the first academic year from an 'A' to a 'C' stream, or from the 'B' stream to the 'C' stream and then fell to the lower half of it. This definition of a deteriorator excluded those who fell from an 'A' to a 'B' stream and also those who were placed in the 'C' stream on entrance. This arbitrary definition was used in the first place in a small scale enquiry in order to provide some objective criterion of deterioration which would isolate those who failed to justify their selection in the entrance examination. Those pupils who fell from the 'A' to the 'B' stream could not be placed in this category. When it was realised that it would be profitable to extend the scale of the work it was then too late to obtain the necessary details for the additional deteriorators.

In Year 5 there was a four-form entry and we added to the deteriorators those who had fallen by the end of the first academic year from the 'C' stream to the 'D' stream and found a low position in that stream, together with pupils who had fallen from higher streams. We accepted the limitations of this definition because we wished to examine the causes of deterioration rather than to determine its incidence. The definition adopted ensured that deteriorators were those whose standard of work fell so sharply during their first year in the grammar school that they caused concern to the school authorities.

A Personal Approach

The deteriorators when found were studied individually. Each deteriorator was given Schonell tests in word recognition and diagnostic arithmetic, and intelligence tests. The results of

4

several intelligence tests were available for other pupils in addition to those for deteriorators. Primary school records were scrutinised and checked for absenteeism and ill-health; the Principal School Medical Officer for the County was asked for the health-grading of each deteriorator; home background and outside-school behaviour were probed; a record card for each was filled in and 'favourite subjects', 'subjects disliked most', outside-school activities and so on, duly ascertained and recorded. The Probation Officer was consulted in cases of known misdemeanour and her knowledge sought about all the deteriorators. Headteachers, teachers, youth leaders and Ministers of Religion were also interviewed. The home of each deteriorator was visited at least once and on occasion more than once when a previous impression needed checking.

It was found, as might be expected, that deteriorators originated from all types of primary schools and were scattered over a wide area. Although each case was investigated in some detail, it was considered that more light would be shed on the problem if a closer investigation was undertaken in an area based on one particular primary school. This school was selected because it produced a much higher proportion of deteriorators than did other schools. Here the chief problem appeared to be whether deterioration was due to the type of instruction in the primary school, or to the character of the homes in its catchment area. The account of this section of the enquiry is given in another chapter.

Character of the Grammar School

The co-educational grammar school where these studies were made is situated in a small industrial area with an agricultural background. It had a three-form entry in Years 1, 2, 3 and 4, and a four-form entry in Year 5. The intake into the school has varied from about 39 per cent of the relevant age-group in Year 3, to about 46 per cent in Year 4. In Year 1, 2 and 5 the percentage intake varied between the limits of 39 per cent and 46 per cent. These percentages are high and will be commented upon later.

An indication of the social class to which the children entering the school belonged is given in Table 1. The categories

1–7 are based on the classification adopted by Glass[1]. The sample consists of the entire entry for one year. It was compiled from information gathered from each pupil about the precise occupation of the father.

TABLE I
Classification by Parental Occupation

Category	1	2	3	4	5	6	7
No. of pupils[2]	6	9	10	9	41	21	6
% of pupils	5·9	8·8	9·8	8·8	40·2	20·6	5·9

It will be seen from Table 1 that some 61 per cent of the pupils came from homes where the fathers belonged to Categories 5 and 6, i.e. the skilled manual and semi-skilled manual classes.

The categories of occupation in Table 1 are as follows:—

1. Professional and High Administrative, e.g. Medical Officer, Company Director, Chartered Accountant, Solicitor.
2. Managerial and Executive, e.g. Personnel Manager, Headmaster (elem.), Civil Servant (executive class), Business Manager, Nonconformist Minister, Farmer.
3. Inspectional, Supervisory and other Non-Manual e.g. Police Inspector, Elementary School Teacher, Jobbing Master, Builder, Reporter, Commercial Traveller.
4. As for 3 but lower grade, e.g. Costing Clerk, Relieving Officer, Chef, Insurance Agent, Newsagent and Tobacconist.
5. Skilled Manual and routine grades of Non-Manual e.g. Fitter, Routine Clerk, Carpenter, Policeman, Shop Assistant.
6. Semi-skilled Manual e.g. Tractor Driver, Railway Porter, Agricultural Labourer, Carter.
7. Unskilled Manual e.g. Dock Labourer, Road Sweeper, Watchman.

More than half the pupils came from homes connected with some aspect of engineering; a substantial percentage were connected with business (mainly shops); then came farming, the military services and the 'white collars', in that order.

[1] Glass, D. V. edited by, *Social Mobility in Britain*, London, 1954.
[2] This is the number of pupils who actually entered the first form in that year; some did not complete the year.

The School and the Problem

In addition to examination results, there was also available for each entrant an assessment of home background by the Head Teachers of the junior school. The analysis of these assessments showed however, that they were far from sufficiently reliable for our purposes. As it had become clear that much additional information about the homes was needed, we then decided, as mentioned previously, to make an independent assessment of home influence by visiting the homes of as many deteriorators as possible. In addition, a special investigation was undertaken of the home background of pupils in a particular Junior School, which shall be known as 'School X'. The homes of some improvers were also visited.

The Entrance Examination

In the entrance examinations of Years 1, 2 and 3 the subjects were English (mainly comprehension), Arithmetic (mental, mechanical and problems), and an Intelligence Test. In Years 4 and 5 the examination was changed, and consisted of a standardised English test with one essay and two short descriptions, which were marked subjectively on a percentage basis, a standardised Arithmetic test and an Intelligence test. This variation in the entrance examination from year to year might lead us to regard any deductions with respect to academic deterioration open to a wide range of errors. But our definition of deteriorators is severe enough to leave no doubt in our minds about their classification. Moreover all the deteriorators were sufficiently high in the entrance examination lists to make us reasonably confident that they would have entered the grammar school if they had taken either of these examinations.

II

APTITUDE AND ATTAINMENT

BY some merciful provision of Providence children are different
from each other, intellectually as well as in other ways. They
differ in their inborn ability to reason, they differ in the
environments which equip this reasoning ability for action, they
differ in their desire to use this ability in various situations.
They are also far from equal in many other intellectual abilities.
For example some are gifted in the use of numbers, others in
handling words, others in perceiving relationship between
shapes and between diagrams, and so on. These are the type
of intellectual abilities which are needed for success in work of
an academic type, and the most important of them, for our
purpose, is the ability to reason. We therefore made an early
examination of this factor in both the deteriorators and the
control group.

Intelligence or Academic Aptitude

The verbal intelligence test is acknowledged to be one of the
best predictors of later academic success. A Working Party of
the British Psychological Society (Vernon, 1957) surveying and
summing up the evidence, came to the conclusion that 'the
usual combination of Intelligence, English and Arithmetic tests
reaches a very high degree of validity (the Intelligence test
being usually the best single predictor)'. The type of intelligence
test referred to is the verbal group type, which was the main
intelligence test used in this study.

At the end of their first academic year group intelligence
tests were administered to all the deteriorators. For a control

8

group of 88 pupils, being a cross-section from all streams, use
was made of the intelligence test taken in the entrance examination. The average I.Q. of the deteriorators was 111·4, and that
for the control group 110·3. It is reasonable to assume from
these figures that the deteriorators as a group were not handicapped by being of lower intelligence than their fellow pupils.
The I.Q. range of the deteriorators was as follows—

TABLE 2

I.Q.	No. of Deteriorators
130+	—
125–129	—
120–124	3
115–119	6
110–114	13
105–109	15
100–104	2
Below 100	—

Average I.Q.=111·4

At first sight it might seem that the intelligence level of some
of these deteriorators was rather low for grammar school work
and indeed this factor may have played some part in the
deterioration. In order to throw further light on this problem
we compared the I.Q.s of deteriorators with those of the non-
deteriorators of the same sex who were in corresponding
positions in the same entrance examination. We were able to
do this for Years 4 and 5 of the survey, comprising only 14 of
the deteriorators, but we found that whereas the average I.Q.
of the deteriorators was 112·9, that of the non-deteriorators was
only 110·2. We see therefore that pupils who had the same or
slightly lower I.Q.s than the deteriorators did not themselves
become deteriorators. This indicates, as one would expect, that
factors other than intelligence have a strong influence on
academic success. In the clinical case study work we came
across only two pupils where we concluded that lack of ability
was the principal factor associated with deterioration, though
there were two other cases where it was a strong contributory
factor.

Data gathered from other sections of the enquiry point in the
same direction. We have already said by implication that no

deteriorator by the demotion definition could come from the pupils who were in the bottom thirty in the entrance examination. This bottom group represented a third of the pupils for the first four years and a quarter for the fifth year. In addition the lowest placed deteriorator for all five years was no lower than 62nd out of 113 acceptancies for Year 5. The other lowest placed deteriorators were 61st out of 103 in Year 1, 58th out of 94 in Year 2, 47th out of 78 in Year 3 and 54th out of 95 in Year 4. Many pupils who were placed in a lower position in the entrance examination did not deteriorate and did creditable work.

In the same connection we examined the junior school assessment of these pupils in comparison with that for other pupils. The information was obtained for Years 2, 3 and 4 and Table 3 shows the assessment of all pupils in these years. Group 1 gives those pupils considered by the teachers to possess the ability and aptitude for grammar school education, Group 2 those who were border-line, and Group 3 those who lacked the ability and aptitude for grammar school education.

TABLE 3

Junior School Assessment of Grammar School Candidates[1]

	Group 1		Group 2		Group 3	
Year	No. of pupils	Failed final entrance exam.	No. of pupils	Failed final entrance exam.	No. of pupils	Failed final entrance exam.
2	66	20	48	18	96	92
3	54	16	41	16	102	98
4	51	6	43	20	111	97
	171	42	132	54	309	287

Junior school teachers allocated seven out of 20 deteriorators for these years to the failure group, i.e. Group 3, seven to the border-line group and six to the top group. Readers are reminded, however, that there is a 'ceiling' effect in reverse, by which those pupils placed in the last 30 places in the entrance examination could not become deteriorators under the selected definition. Similarly those pupils who were demoted from the

[1] Some were unobtainable.

'A' to the 'B' stream and dropped no further during the first year were not classed as deteriorators, partly because they might still be regarded as being of reasonable academic standard. We see that six of these 20 deteriorators were classed as having ability and aptitude for grammar school education, and another seven were placed in the middle group with many other pupils who had a successful career at the grammar school. Some of the deteriorators gained really high positions in the entrance examination, e.g. 3rd, 5th, 11th, 12th, 15th, 21st (2 pupils). Summaries of the case studies of many of these pupils will be given at the end of the book.

Attainment Tests

Although a measure of the attainment of the pupils was available in the end-of-year examinations, it was decided that objective tests in English and Arithmetic would possibly throw light on some of the causes of deterioration, as reasonable ability in these subjects is a pre-requisite to success in most of the others. With that end in view, Word Recognition (Schonell, 1946) and Diagnostic Arithmetic Tests (Schonell, 1951) were used. The former was set to each individual deteriorator, following an informal chat on topics of general interest at school and especially about reading material such as books and periodicals read at home. The test was given in the spirit of a challenge and checking of mistakes was made as inconspicuous as possible. There was no suggestion that it was a 'reading test' at any stage.

The Diagnostic Arithmetic Test was given to groups. As not all deteriorators were in the same form (or class) in a given year, it was not possible to avoid forming the deteriorators for the same entrance year into one group for the purpose of the Arithmetic Test. The administrator of the test was, however, satisfied that the motivation of the pupils was good and that they were doing their best.

The principle of gaining the confidence of a pupil (and very often, not only that of the pupil, but of others connected with him or her, such as parents) in a case study approach such as this, cannot be over-estimated. Where there is lack of sympathy with the grammar school and a tendency to revolt against academic discipline, confidence between teacher and pupil is sometimes difficult to establish. We must remember, also, that deteriorators are often emotionally unstable. Schonell (1936) found amongst the backward a disproportionate number of emotionally unstable children; three times as many as amongst those making satisfactory progress. A conscious effort was therefore made to ensure that the child had the right attitude to the work before testing began.

A whole year's entry (101 pupils) was tested with the same Schonell Word Recognition Test as the deteriorators of Years 1 to 5. The testing for both deteriorators and control group was done in their second year of attendance. The range of the Word Reading Quotients of the deteriorators was from 108·1 to 84·9, and only nine of the thirty-nine were over 100. Whereas the average Quotient for deteriorators was 95, that of a normal year's entry was 108·8 for girls and 105·9 for boys. For both girls and boys, the differences between the deteriorators and the pupils who entered in Year 7 (who would themselves contain some future deteriorators) are significant at the 0·1 per cent level of confidence.

The average Word Recognition Quotients for the Year 7 entry—108·8 for girls and 105·9 for boys—were low for grammar school pupils, but this might have been due largely if not entirely to the admission to the school of such a high percentage of the total age group. This relatively low average was of little concern to us, however, as the principal aim was to compare a control group with the deteriorators.

The fact that for both boy and girl deteriorators the average Word Recognition Quotients were much lower (by 12 to 13 points) than for the control group was of some interest in view of the general similarity of deteriorators and controls in test scores of intelligence or academic aptitude, on entry. Though here and there the low Word Recognition Quotient might in part have been due to a wrong emotional attitude during testing—one girl was embarrassingly reserved, another seemed nervous and one boy possibly set up a resistance and did not fully exert himself—the results of the group are in line with the general academic deterioration which brought about their selection as deteriorators. Whatever the reason for their low standard, whether lack of ability or lack of cultural background or lack of interest, these pupils were undoubtedly severely handicapped in their progress in many other subjects by their low standard of reading. When they were admitted to the grammar school their scores in English in relation to their ages were appreciably higher. Although the two tests used do not measure exactly the same abilities, and we would not expect the performance of any single pupil to be necessarily similar for both tests, we would expect some general similarity in the performances of a group taking the two tests. On the contrary, there is a decided difference between the standard of the group in Word Recognition and that in English some two years previously.

The Schonell Diagnostic Arithmetic Tests served to throw a strong light on specific deficiencies. The deteriorators again and again showed lack of care or ignorance of fundamentals. One girl always multiplied wrongly by nought; a boy and another girl were wrong in every sum requiring multiplication by double figures; two other boys had considerable trouble with graded multiplication as well; another made persistent and consistent blunders in his multiplication tables (e.g. $8 \times 7 = 57$), another boy and girl always left out noughts in the answer when dividing (e.g. $1515 \div 5 = 33$). One boy made little real effort even in the test; this attitude was characteristic of the boy—his behaviour was the same in games, woodwork, etc., so that he was finally transferred to a secondary modern school. In every case the Arithmetic score, in relation to age, showed a distinct drop from the score obtained in the entrance examination. What, therefore, may be the cause of such deterioration in arithmetic? Schonell (1940) stresses the importance of the emotional factors. He writes, 'Backwardness in arithmetic is due as much to emotional as to intellectual factors . . . normal emotional reactions are *more important* than normal intellectual ones to arithmetic.' Biggs (1951) summarises the main causes as (1) bad home background, (ii) bad health on the part of the pupil, (iii) absence from school, (iv) numerous changes of staff, and (v) emotional attitude of child to mathematics. In our survey (ii) and (iv) are not conspicuous, but there is evidence for the effect of the other three on some of the deteriorators. These effects are examined in other chapters.

III

THE INFLUENCE OF THE HOME

THROUGHOUT our investigation the relationship between the nature of the home and the attainment of the pupil was frequently and sometimes forcibly brought to our attention. For a long time teachers have been aware of the influence of the home on individual pupils, but the influence's strength and pervasiveness were not fully appreciated. The concept of social class gathers under its umbrella many of the factors in the home which are associated with pupil attainment; it also lends itself easily to objective classification and analysis. We shall begin therefore, with this constellation in general and then deal with some of its component factors. First, however, we should perhaps point out that defective home backgrounds are not the sole prerogative of any one social class, nor are the 'defects' limited to those of a material kind; they clearly include the intellectual and the emotional.

As assessed clinically these defects played a major part in the deterioration of 25 of the 39 deteriorators, contributed substantially to the deterioration of four other pupils, and had a slighter effect on four others. In two other cases, where the home was an asset, there was recovery from deterioration, and one of these eventually even improved on his status at entry. The improvers also were blessed with good homes. In two cases the principal factor in deterioration has been classified as 'emotional upset' and not under 'home background' because, although the cause of the upset may in one way be said to have originated in the home, yet the home could do nothing about it and was otherwise a good home. In one case the child suddenly discovered that he or she was illegitimate and in the other the mother suddenly died at a critical time in the child's career.

Social Class

The association between severe deterioration in attainment and the character of the home was first noticed clinically. The authors therefore prepared a table in which the occupations of the fathers of the pupils were classified for

(a) one whole year of entry
(b) the 'improvers' for Years 1 to 6 inclusive
(c) deteriorators for Years 1 to 5 inclusive.

The improvers included all pupils who conformed to a promotion criterion; they are presented here because they bring the social class factor into even greater prominence. It should be noted that the one year of entry will in itself contain some deteriorators and some improvers.

TABLE 4
Classification for Social Status from Parental Occupation

Parental Occupation Category:	1	2	3	4	5	6	7
No. of pupils—one year	6	9	10	9	41	21	6
No. of improvers—							
Years 1 to 6 inclusive	0	6	7	8	15	0	0
No. of deteriorators—							
Years 1 to 5 inclusive	0	0	0	2	15	12	10

Readers are reminded that Class 1 is professional and high administrative and Class 7 unskilled manual workers.

In the table the deteriorators tend to congregate in the skilled, semi-skilled and unskilled manual working classes, i.e. 37 out of 39 are in these categories; on the other hand the improvers do not go below the skilled manual class[1]. The fathers of 22 of the 39 deteriorators were unskilled or semi-

[1] Statistical comparisons (Chi-square) of the social class distribution of deteriorators compared with the one-year entry (itself 'contaminated' with improvers and deteriorators) gives a significant difference well beyond the ·025 level. The comparison between deteriorators and improvers gave a highly significant difference. That between improvers and the one-year entry was significant beyond the ·05 level. Yates' correction was used in each case.

skilled, i.e. 56·4 per cent, whereas only 26·5 per cent of the pupils in a whole year's entry (including future deteriorators) belonged to these classes. This finding is confirmed by other researches, notably the Ministry of Education report 'Early Leaving', page 18, where it is stated that:—

'deterioration which has caused many who were placed in the top selection group at eleven, to be found at sixteen in the lowest academic categories, is most common among the children of unskilled workers (54 per cent) and semi-skilled workers (37·9 per cent).'

At the other end of the table none of the 39 cases of deterioration gathered from five years of entry, came from the professional, executive and inspectional classes, whereas 13 out of the 36 improvers came from these classes. Even in the middle of the scale, Class 4, or the lower supervisory workers, contains eight out of the 36 improvers but only two out of the 39 deteriorators.

In an attempt to isolate more specifically the particular influences associated with deterioration we included a detailed examination of a number of factors in the social class 'constellation'. Our findings on two factors appear to be of special significance and are treated more fully than the others, on which we have less conclusive evidence. The first of these is the education of the parents.

Parental Education

We began with a control group consisting of the total entry for two years and tabulated the pupils according to stream and education of parents. This information is given in Table 5.

TABLE 5
Streaming in relation to education of parents (Percentages)[1]

	'A' stream	'B' stream	'C' stream
Number of children (Years 7 and 8)	64	63	54
(a) No parent attended grammar school	15·1	31·5	53·4
(b) Only mother attended grammar school	32·3	38·7	29·0
(c) Only father attended grammar school	51·2	39·5	9·3
(d) Both parents attended grammar school	61·8	32·4	5·9

[1] The difference between (a) and (b) is significant beyond the ·05 level, and those between (a) and (c), and between (a) and (d) beyond the ·001 level.

There were 108 families out of 181 with one or more parents who were taught at a grammar school. It should be noted in passing that whereas 83 per cent of children in the 'A' stream had at least one parent who was educated in a grammar school, this proportion declined to 63 per cent in the 'B' form and only 28 per cent in the 'C' form. (Cf. Whalley (1961) pp. 138–140, and pp. 45–57). From these figures alone one cannot say that the differences are produced solely by a decline in parental encouragement, as such factors as the correlation between social class and academic aptitude are also involved. The case study evidence, however, on progress in the grammar school, points strongly to parental influence as a major factor. The differences are most pronounced when both parents attended a grammar school, and when only the father attended a grammar school. When only the mother attended a grammar school the differences, as shown in the Table, do not appear as great, but one would not care to make a definite finding from a single instance and with such small numbers. (Cf. Douglas, 1964, p. 43).

We then examined the parental education of the deteriorators and found to our surprise that in *only one case amongst the 39 was there a parent educated in a grammar school*, whereas we have seen that in the control sample of a one-year entry there were 108 out of 181 families with one or more parents who were taught at a grammar school[1]. The research of Jones (1962) gives general support to these findings. His research produced a statistically significant association between deterioration and neither of the parents having been educated at a grammar school, and between deterioration and the mother not having been educated at a grammar school, but the difference caused by the father not receiving a grammar school education was not statistically significant, though the trend was the same. Further support for the influence of the mother on the educational progress of the child comes from our examination of the parental education of the full 36 improvers discovered in the entries of Years 1 to 6. Both the parents of one third of the improvers were educated at a grammar school, only the mothers of another third (30·6 per cent) were so educated, and in the case of 19·4 per cent of improvers only the father was so

[1] The difference is statistically highly significant.

educated. In only 16·6 per cent of the cases did neither parent attend a grammar school. We are supported in this finding by the work of Greenald (1955), who concluded that there was some association between improvement and the parents' further or grammar school education[1].

The scarcity of grammar-school parents amongst the deteriorators does not, of course, imply an inevitable lack of academic culture in the home; but it does mean that all these parents have missed the experience of grammar school life and studies which could help them with their children's difficulties; and it cannot be easy for them to understand fully what the school requires of them as parents. Lewis (1952) writes '. . . it was often more difficult for a boy from a poorer home to 'fit in' as naturally as a boy whose parents had been to grammar schools, and where their own backgrounds and interests were not unlike those of the schoolmasters the boy would meet in school.' Thus in seven cases of the 39 there was evidence of the reading of light novels by one or both parents, the other parents read newspapers and periodicals only. Another survey, reported in 'Allocation Studies No. 5' (1955) of the National Foundation for Educational Research, has similar findings. It gives the results of interviews with 191 parents in a suburb of London; it states that '. . . reading at the level of illustrated and feature magazines was related positively to improvement (22) and reading at the level of comics and women's papers to deterioration (31). For two-thirds of the sample, the type of newspaper taken in the home was approximately independent of trend of achievement; although in a small group where no paper at all was taken, there was a trend towards deterioration'.

A number of researches have now demonstrated this finding, e.g. Metcalfe (1950, p. 63): 'The provision of (good) books in the home proved a significant factor' (for academic progress). Fraser (1959) pp. 43–46, comes to the same conclusion.

The second factor selected was size of family.

Family Size

While we were examining the association between family poverty and deterioration in attainment we came across

---

[1] Cf. also the important book by Fraser, E. (1959) pp. 41–43.

important differences concerning family size. This is an aspect of the question which merits much more attention. As Stott (1956) states: 'When one examines the home background of delinquents or even of children who are backward at school, one cannot help remarking how frequently they are members of large families, and recent studies confirm that the numbers coming from such families are indeed disproportionate.' Even when social class is held constant, this effect of family size can be seen at work. (Cf. Floud *et al*, Table 21).

Not only is a large family more likely to draw near the poverty line, and therefore, be unable to pay for facilities such as books and the comfort of a fire for homework, but also interruption by other children in the family may help substantially towards the deterioration of a grammar school pupil. Four of our deteriorators suffered badly from such interruptions. Nor can the parents give as much attention to any one of five or six children as they could to an only child.

The difference between the size of the families of the deteriorators and those of a control group is shown in Table 6

TABLE 6

Size of Family

Number of children in family

	6 or more %	5 %	4 %	3 %	2 %	1 %
One-year entry (95 pupils not counting deteriorators)	—	8·7	21·7	17·4	39·1	13·0
Deteriorators in the Survey (39) (Years 1 to 5)	18·0	5·1	28·2	15·4	20·5	12·8

This table was prepared by noting the number of children in the family of each deteriorator, towards the end of the pupil's first year of attendance.

It will be seen that whereas 51 per cent of the deteriorators belonged to families where there were four or more children, only 30 per cent of the non-deteriorators were similarly placed and in the entry year considered in Table 6 there was no family of a non-deteriorator which had more than five children. The average size of the families of deteriorators was 3·9 whereas that of the 36 improvers was 2·1. Greenald (1955) came to the same conclusion. He reported that a family size of four children or more was associated with a downward trend in academic performance, in both middle and working classes. Academic improvement was associated with only children, particularly among the working class. In this study 67 per cent of the improvers were the first-born of a small family; the figure for deteriorators was 48·7 per cent.[1]

In order to ascertain more clearly the inter-relationship between social class, size of family and pupil attainment the data was reorganised as it appears in Table 7.

TABLE 7

Size of Family and Social Class
Deteriorators compared with Improvers[a]

Children in Family		Social Class					
		2	3	4	5	6	7
1	Deteriorators				2	2	1
	Improvers	(1)	(4)	(3)	(5)		
2	Deteriorators			1	1	3	3
	Improvers		(3)	(3)	(7)		
3	Deteriorators				3	2	1
	Improvers	(4)		(2)	(1)		
4	Deteriorators			1	4	2	4
	Improvers				(2)		
5	Deteriorators				1	1	
	Improvers						
6	Deteriorators				2	1	
	Improvers						
More than 6	Deteriorators				2	1	1
	Improvers	(1)					

[1] The differences are statistically significant.

[a] Improvers are in brackets; they are from Years 1 to 6, whereas deteriorators are from Years 1 to 5.

The dotted line is drawn to include all but one of the 36 improvers. When one reads from left to right, there are no improvers below social class 5 (skilled manual) and when one reads downwards there is only one improver from families of more than 4 children. In this exceptional case the father was a professional man (social class 2). Within each social class the family size of the improvers is smaller than that of the deteriorators; in social class 4 (lower supervisory) it is 1·9 compared with 3·0 and in social class 5 (skilled manual) it is 2·0 compared with 4·9. The other classes do not overlap, but for social class 3 (supervisory) the average size for improvers was 1·4, and in social class 2 (executive) it was 3·6 (because of the exceptional family of 9); for deteriorators in class 6 (semi-skilled) the average size was 3·6 and for those in class 7 (unskilled) 3·4. As the number of deteriorators was only 39, and there were only 36 improvers, we record this information mainly to enable comparisons to be made with the results of other investigations.

Once again, however, we feel it necessary to remind readers of the 'floor' and 'ceiling' effects due to our definition of improvers and deteriorators. A large proportion of the higher social class children were in the 'A' stream on entry, because of their high place in the entrance examination. They were therefore more 'at risk' than those from the lower social classes, except that they were not included as deteriorators if they went down only to the 'B' stream. Pupils in the 'A' stream could not, however, become improvers. On the other hand there was a large proportion of pupils of low social class in the lowest stream. It was therefore statistically easier for them to produce improvers, whereas they could not, by definition, become deteriorators. Our working definitions, therefore, tend to produce an underestimate of the association between social class and attainment in the grammar school.

In the remaining sections of this chapter we present evidence on other aspects of the home background, without, however, being able to compare it with evidence derived from a control group of pupils who made normal progress. Lacking the necessary financial resources and manpower we were unable to do this. Though we visited the homes of some of the improvers, the visits were too few to afford an adequate basis for statistical comparison. None the less we present the results here because we consider that they are interesting, and valuable as clinical evidence.

Home Facilities

One of the most obvious differences between the social classes, for our purposes, is in the facilities—or handicaps—which help or hinder the pupil while doing homework. Though this provision is sometimes merely a reflection of the attitude of the parents towards education, and the priority which they give to other things, such as radio, television and entertaining, it is often largely determined by limitations of accommodation and by finance. Its importance is illustrated by the finding of one research worker (Metcalfe, 1950) that those factors which do influence school progress are such as affect homework facilities. We ourselves found that in 20 of the 39 homes of deteriorators there was normally no fire in any room other than the kitchen or living-room, and in nine of these cases there was also fairly constant interruption from other members of the family, mainly children. One of these and another pupil (aged 11 plus) were regularly kept in charge of their youngest brothers and sisters for the evening. The industrious type of child would often triumph over these difficulties, but not all children are industrious. While interviewing the parents in the homes the visitor became acutely aware that almost always it is not one single factor which is responsible for a pupil's lack of progress, but an interacting combination of factors, though one or two major factors are often clearly discernible.

There is a suggestion in *Early Leaving* (1954) p. 40, for assisting boys and girls who have poor opportunities for doing homework, viz:—

> Boys and girls who had poor facilities for doing homework at their own home might be accommodated after school hours at (a) the grammar school, or (b) the primary school which they attended before entering the grammar school, or (c) some other convenient centre, e.g. Public Library, Youth Club.

Suggestion (b) would have been helpful in thirteen 'cases' of this survey; the others were far removed from the suggested facilities. If they could have stayed at the grammar school after the afternoon session, eleven local 'cases' would have benefited; suggestion (c) would have been difficult in this area because of lack of accommodation.

It is heartening to see that in Bootle since 1955 'a new branch library includes a successful children's homework centre equipped with study carrels, individual desk lights and a plentiful stock of reference books'. Similar experiments are being tried in other large cities.

In most regions the presence of a television set in the only room where there is a fire increases the handicap of the working class child compared with the child of a professional or executive father. The problem has been so serious in some cases as to impel the Head to send a circular letter to parents asking for their co-operation in ensuring that children are enabled to do their homework in a warm room, without interruption. Other Heads have made the request at Speech Day or through a Parents Association.

Poverty

Lack of money does not, of itself, produce unstable academic performers. There was, however, as we have already seen, a deterioration of an undue proportion of the grammar school children of working class families; in this deterioration the financial factor sometimes played its part. For example, two boy deteriorators had been told early in their school life by one or both of their parents that the financial state of their family could not keep them at school beyond the minimum age for leaving. Both of these boys worked for money in the evenings and on Saturdays. Another boy was possibly conscious of the financial struggle at home; he used to buy his own clothes with his wages as errand boy. There was financial stress, also, at the homes of an additional two boys, so that they took paid 'errand' work at an early stage in their grammar school career.

Financial difficulties also produce premature and early leaving, even though a maintenance grant is given to parents of children who remain at school after their fifteenth birthday. Two of our girl deteriorators because of the more or less

C

permanent illness of the father (though their mother was working) considered their financial position very carefully, did not find the grant sufficient, and left school. But there is no evidence to show that, even if the grant had been doubled in value, these and the other deteriorators who were premature and early leavers would have remained at school. This aspect of early leaving is emphasised in a Report of the Association of Education Committees (1952): 'The amount and incidence of maintenance allowance play an insignificant part'. The Report continues: 'The chief attraction to the early leaver is undoubtedly the money to be received from entering paid employment'.

Another factor, of which readers should be reminded, is that within each social class, deteriorators tend to come from larger families; it is by no means unlikely that financial difficulties played a part here.

Other research also shows the influence of financial stringency. Ault (1940) concludes that 'unemployment or casual employment of father' is one of six causes of backwardness in secondary school work. Fraser (1959) pp. 46–49, working in Aberdeen, also found poverty to have an appreciable effect, even when intelligence level had been taken into account.

Further evidence of the impact of poverty on scholastic progress is provided by the National Foundation for Educational Research, Allocation Study, No. 5, 1955. It states: 'Where there has been financial difficulty there is a trend towards deterioration . . .'; further: 'That being an only child is likely to be associated with improvement, especially among the working class pupils, and that belonging to a family of four or more is more likely to be associated with improvement or deterioration than with progress at the predicted level'.

Parental Attitude

We include a short section on parental attitude to the pupil's education because we consider it to be of central importance. Disappointingly, however, we have little new evidence to offer. This is because we were convinced that the only reliable method of obtaining direct and reasonably valid information was by interviewing the parents of *all* the entrants before they had been more than a few months at the grammar school. Only at this stage would the attitudes of the parents be unaffected by the progress—or lack of progress—of their offspring. Later on the encouraging attitude of the parents—if it existed at all—might be undermined by the persistent failures of the deteriorators, while the support of the parents of successful pupils would be strengthened. Our resources were quite inadequate for interviewing on this extensive scale, and we therefore offer only some indirect evidence, and quote a few findings from other sources.

The most obvious indication of parental encouragement of academic progress is seen when parents give high priority to the provision of good facilities for quiet study and homework. This is a first essential, and a good test where the parents are financially able to make the provision. We have seen that in 20 of the deteriorators' homes no fire was provided in a separate room for studying. This was so from the time a fire was first needed in the autumn, so here there is no 'backwash' effect of a pupil's failure. Most of the parents could have afforded this expense if they had seen the necessity of it and adjusted their priorities.

The parents, of course, need to give much more than facilities; constant encouragement—even in the face of failure—is needed. This is much more likely to occur if parents themselves have attended a grammar school and realise what is required of the child, and have a practical insight into the part which they themselves need to play. In our study only one of the 78 parents of the deteriorators had attended a grammar school, and the case studies given later contain plenty of evidence of parental ignorance about homework requirements, of lack of discipline regarding homework, of too frequent attendance at the cinema and social functions, and so on. The parental attitude is also reflected by the premature and early leaving of the deteriorators. Out of eleven deteriorators of the Year 1 entries, nine left without sitting for the Ordinary Level of the G.C.E.; out of seven deteriorators of the Year 2 entries, four left after three years at the Grammar School; and three more left without sitting for a G.C.E. It is realised, as mentioned above, that the lack of success would, in itself, be an incentive to the parent to withdraw the child (cf. Dale, 1957). Collins

25

(1955) also emphasises the waste involved in this premature leaving: '. . . decrease (of premature leaving) requires primarily the development of certain attitudes towards continued education rather than the refinements of selection techniques and the adjustment of grammar school places'. There must be an attitude of mind in the parents which takes for granted the continuation of the child's study as far as the 'Ordinary Level' of the G.C.E., and possibly beyond.

The 'Early Leaving' Report (1954) shows in Table 20 that 24 per cent of the number of girls leaving school prematurely did so because only the parents wished it; 40 per cent left because only the pupils wished it . . . and one wonders how much influence the parents' attitude had on this 40 per cent. The investigation by Floud *et al* (1957, p. 80) adds further evidence. 'The (grammar) schools may find that one in seven (in Middlesbrough) and one in twelve (South-west Hertfordshire) of the children admitted each year (regardless of social origin) are handicapped by the likelihood that their parents will withdraw them at the age of fifteen and the certainty that their parents will not resist any inclination on the children's part to leave school at this age. They may also have to face the fact that approximately another one in four in South-west Hertfordshire and one in three in Middlesbrough will be in the same position at the age of sixteen'. Though premature leaving (i.e. before taking the General Certificate at Ordinary Level) and early leaving (before taking a Sixth Form course) have both been reduced since these figures were published, and reflect a change in public opinion and parental attitude, there is still a long way to go.

Disharmony in the Home

The evidence for harmony or discord in a home is often circumstantial and sometimes hearsay. Very few parents show mutual repugnance before a visitor. Although the field worker visited the homes of the deteriorators and knew the children well, we cannot be at all certain that we have included every instance of serious discord. Our cases are limited to those of a more serious type which cannot be concealed. But in ten cases out of thirty-nine, there is convincing evidence of the psychological turmoil produced in some children by disharmony in the home. These included indisputable records of serious discord in the families of two boy deteriorators just before their entrance to the grammar school, with disastrous effects on their work; another had a father who was physically vicious especially when drunk; the parents of a girl deteriorator were unmarried, and the father was morally unstable and often drunk; the illness of the father was the cause of unfortunate relationships at another boy's home; yet another boy had a home life which can only be described as 'tempestuous'; we have similar incontestable evidence of pronounced discord in another four cases. Further evidence of the same kind is provided by one sixth-form pupil, who was a brilliant student up to the sixth form and then had a serious psychological upset on account of a difficult relationship with one of the parents and also between the parents themselves. The student was persuaded to move from the home to 'digs'. This resulted in a marked recovery and the student managed to pass in two advanced subjects and went on to do well at the university.

We are aware that the evidence would have been strengthened if the homes of the deteriorators had been compared with those of the non-deteriorators, but the difficulty of obtaining satisfactory evidence prevented this being done. However, on the clinical level, the case study material points to disharmony in the home as a far from negligible factor in the production of deteriorators. It would indeed be surprising if this were not so. Other researchers have similar findings. Metcalfe (1950) also found that emotional disturbance is detrimental to school progress. She suggests that the uncooperative parent not only makes no effort to provide conditions and materials for home study or for physical well-being, but by his indifference, or even opposition to the demands made by the school, subjects the child to conflict and frustration and so sets up the state of emotional disturbance which is a significant factor in hindering scholastic and personality success. Fraser (1959, pp. 60–64) also found that an abnormal home background was important in lowering the attainment level, even when intelligence had been allowed for.

There are, however, cases where deterioration does not occur under these circumstances. We have in mind one pupil whose home conditions, well known to the investigator, were far from ideal—the father having a decidedly irresponsible attitude to his home. The child had a stong desire for university education, a factor which enabled her to pursue her studies with commendable single-mindedness; but it must be admitted that the mother was a better influence than the father.

Emotional Disturbance

It is, of course, difficult and often impossible to separate this factor from the home background. We did, however, find five cases where the emotional disturbances did not appear to be produced by disharmony, poverty, or lack of facilities in the home. These severe disturbances were due to a girl's sexual precocity, a boy's discovery of his illegitimacy, the temperamental unbalance of a boy (leading later to confirmed serious illness), the death of a girl's mother, and the prolonged and difficult illness at home of a boy's father. These emotional factors contributed substantially, in our opinion, to the academic deterioration of all five pupils, but in only three of them did it appear to be the principal factor. There is no 'proof', in the scientific sense, that this is so; one is merely making a judgment from the data.

Comment

The evidence presented in this chapter has demonstrated the cardinal importance of a good supporting home background for the satisfactory academic progress of children. While conducting the case studies and while examining the evidence we have been impressed by the frequency with which a child suffers not merely from one handicap in the home but from an accumulation of them. John, who is the son of an unskilled manual labourer has several younger brothers and sisters, and lives in a small house in a poor neighbourhood where the attitude to education is by no means as favourable as elsewhere. There is not enough money to pay for a second fire, there is no second living-room in which homework could be done, and there is no table in a bedroom either. John does his homework in the crowded living-room on the edge of the table, subject to frequent interruptions from other children. If he experiences difficulties in the work he is unable to call in help from his parents. If his homework is unfinished when father or mother want to listen to the radio or to watch television, he either finishes it under difficulties or gives up the struggle. His parents do not know whether the work is finished or not, nor do they show any particular interest. Sometimes John is left in charge of the younger children while his parents have a night out at the pub or the cinema. Sometimes a gang of his friends, who are all at the secondary modern school and have little or no homework, come and tempt John to go out and play before his own work is completed. They perhaps go to the cinema together twice a week. When John is put into a lower stream at the end of the first term at the grammar school, neither parent thinks of going to see the Headmaster to discuss John's deterioration, or if they do think of it, they cannot summon up the initiative or courage to do it. John leaves early because he is 'doing no good at school', the family needs his earnings, and his friends are leaving the secondary modern school and flinging their money about on girl friends and bicycles while John has 2/6 a week pocket money and—no girl friend.

On the other hand David is the son of professional parents who have themselves been educated in a grammar school. They provide him with facilities for doing homework in a separate room and light a fire when necessary. There is therefore little interruption from other members of the family or from television and radio. If he has trouble with his homework he can turn to either his mother or father for help, and many books of reference are available. His cultural background is constantly a help to him at school and in his homework. Mother or father may even inspect his homework regularly or occasionally. If he appears to be losing ground his parents arrange an interview with the Headmaster to discuss the matter. If he is absent from school for a long period the parents arrange for a tutor to visit the home to give special help with subjects such as English and Mathematics. David's friends all expect to be at school till they are 18 and many of them expect to go on to a university. David also receives a lot of attention from his parents because there are only a few children in the family. He himself aims high in order to do at least as well as his parents, and his parents encourage him to do so[1].

Not all working class pupils are as badly off as John and not all pupils of professional class parents are as well off as David, but the trends are there, and to endeavour to hide them would do a real disservice to the working classes themselves. It has become axiomatic that educational progress depends greatly on social reform.

[1] Cf. 'Education under Social Handicap', Report on Education No. 17, Department of Education and Science, London, December 1964.

IV

OTHER INFLUENCES

THERE are a multitude of influences which affect the attainment of a pupil at school. In the previous chapters we have considered the ability and attainment of the deteriorator in relation to his fellow pupils, and the nature of his home. We now come to various other influences, each of which has its importance, but to none of which we wish to devote more than a section of a chapter. The first of these is about certain aspects of the personality of the deteriorator himself.

Personal Qualities

It is surprisingly sometimes forgotten that a main factor associated with deterioration lies in the pupil's own personality. So far the home has been the villain of the piece, but the child himself plays his own part. You may lead an unwilling horse to the water, but you cannot make him drink; you may place a child at a desk but you cannot be certain that he is working satisfactorily. Sometimes, as we have seen, the parents may neglect to place the child at the desk. Sometimes, also, the temperamental qualities of the child himself can produce a diminution in parental encouragement or maybe a persistent recrimination which exacerbates the child's undesirable temperamental qualities, and may create an even greater detestation of school work, thus creating a vicious downward spiral which is most difficult to reverse.

The most important temperamental quality the child needs for academic advancement is persistence or industriousness. But the degree of persistence shown by a child in the junior school may change markedly after he enters the grammar school. In the former school the child is under pressure from a teacher whose reputation is seriously affected by the performance of his pupils in the eleven-plus examination; in the latter the pressure on the teacher and to a lesser degree on the pupil is released until it builds up again years later for the next external examination. The situation is very different and the proportion of time spent on homework increases this difference.

The factors causing lack of persistence are peculiar to each individual: if they are not innate they may be due to parental influence, social distraction, or lack of vocational urge. McIntosh (1948) mentions some others—'. . . desire to take up work, unsuitable secondary course, change of school, and changes in health and personal qualities after enrolment in a secondary course'.

Of the 39 deteriorators in this survey, only five were said to be 'persevering' by their junior school head teacher. But in their first year at the grammar school even they, like most other deteriorators, could gain no more than a 'D' for persistence, from the form teacher, on a five-point scale. This was in contrast to the improvers, who obtained a 'B' or 'C' for persistence in their first year. It may be that the five pupils were noticeably persistent in the junior school because of the effort they made in preparation for the entrance examination to the grammar school. But one of them, according to the junior school report, only showed persistence when encouraged in his efforts; once inside the grammar school he slackened off.

After weighing up each case carefully we considered that in nine of the 39 the principal factor associated with deterioration was 'temperamental qualities' and of these by far the most important was lack of persistence. We included under this sub-heading only those children who were thought to be themselves responsible for the absence of effort. There were often, of course, other contributory factors. With 17 other children this lack of persistence was itself a contributory factor, the principal factor being something else such as inadequate parental discipline or emotional disharmony in the home. It is noticeable that both when lack of persistence was the principal cause and when it was contributory, the boys had a greater proportion of cases than did the girls. This would be expected from general psychological theory.

Other Influences

Sometimes the lack of persistence at school work was obviously due to a great liking for doing something else! There were six out of 39 'cases' whose interest in games and sports took their minds off the academic work. One of them is included in the nine for whom the low level of persistence was considered to be the principal cause of their poor attainment. Five of them were passionately fond of hockey or football, while one boy was over-fond of cricket. We do not of course imply by this comment that sports in themselves produce deteriorators: on the contrary, sports are an essential contribution to character building. Everything depends on the pupil securing a proper balance between sports and studies. Another boy undoubtedly spent too many out-of-school hours tinkering with his father's motor bike. Another had a passion for modelling aeroplanes and testing them out, while one of the girls later in her school career spent much of her time with her boy friend (not a pupil of the school) and soon left school to get married. But it must be admitted that those who had a handwork hobby talked enthusiastically about their activities at home and, no doubt, derived much benefit from them.

Our numbers were too small for drawing conclusions about the influence of various types of out-of-school interests on academic deterioration. We were not persuaded that attending cinemas was a major cause of deterioration in this survey; and we had not enough evidence to support Lewis (1952) that 'poor achievers had a tendency to favour outdoor activities, namely a group of four—football, watching football, swimming and cycling'. The largest single out-of-school activity amongst deteriorators was concerned with youth movements, including Church organisations, to which seven girls and eight boys were affiliated. It is our experience that 'club evenings' can be beneficial to youthful members, such as the first year pupils of grammar schools, when used with moderation; but there was evidence that some of the fifteen deteriorators who were active members of clubs regarded them as an 'evening out' with consequent neglect of school work.

Ill-Health and Absence

It would seem self-evident that the academic progress of a child would depend substantially on him remaining in good physical health. In practice the great majority of boys and girls are usually in reasonably good health, so that this factor is not as powerful as a number of others. We thought it essential, however, to get some facts on this point.

A health grading was available for every pupil at entrance to the grammar school. The grades were in three categories:—

Grade A: Excellent general condition.

Grade B: Average or normal condition.

Grade C: Poor physical condition.

According to the Principal School Medical Officer 'C' was the grading which might interfere with academic progress. A normal, healthy person, or one with a minor ailment, such as swollen tonsils, was graded 'B'.

TABLE 8

Medical Grades

	Grade A	Grade B	Grade C
One year's entry (112)[1]	(46) 41·1%	(66) 58·9%	0
Deteriorators[2] (36)	(10) 27·8%	(26)72·2%	0
All secondary schools in the County	12·2%	86·0%	1·8%

If we compare the health grades of the deteriorators in the Table with that of the pupils from one year's entry, the deteriorators *in this sample* have a somewhat lower grading. We know, however, that the deteriorators are on the average of lower social class than the remaining pupils, and that lower social class pupils tend to get rather lower health gradings than the average, whether they are deteriorators or not. Moreover, the smallness of the difference between the deteriorators and the normal entry is demonstrated clearly if we transfer only four deteriorators from medical grade 'B' to medical grade 'A'; the deteriorators then have the same proportions as the normal entry. Not one of the deteriorators had a 'C' category. We can conclude that bad health was not a widespread cause of deterioration in this study. This is not to deny that poor health can and does cause some deterioration in academic studies. The National Foundation for Educational Research in Alloca-

[1] Includes deteriorators and improvers.

[2] Medical grades for three deteriorators not known.

tion Studies No. 5 found that 'poor or indifferent health was positively related to academic deterioration'.

Even in this study there were pupils with minor defects which handicapped their progress at school. Two girl and two boy deteriorators had defective eyesight and had been prescribed spectacles; but they preferred not to wear them. Another girl had very weak eyesight and another boy was slightly deaf. Clearly these six deteriorators must have been handicapped by the above difficulties. Unfortunately we have no evidence about other pupils who may have had similar difficulties but who overcame them and did not lose ground.

Absence from school, whether caused by ill-health or other reasons, inevitably affects academic progress, and as would be expected a number of the deteriorators had poor attendance records. Four of them were particularly affected. One boy took 95 half-days off in the second and third terms of the first year, playing truant without the knowledge of his parents, and two boys and a girl were absent for periods of about 60 half-days, only one of them having a long illness. There were seven others who were away from school for over 40 half-days for often inadequate reasons. Most of the absences, however, were not in the first term, and as deterioration had invariably started by the end of that term, the absences may have been not so much the cause as the result of academic difficulties and failure. They would, however, tend to prevent a recovery.

In view of the above figures it is somewhat surprising to find that the average percentage attendance of deteriorators, however, was very similar to that of all other pupils in corresponding years. For the five years of our Survey, the average percentage attendances are given:—

TABLE 9

	Year 1	Year 2	Year 3	Year 4	Year 5
For deteriorators	89·5%	90·0%	93·2%	93·9%	92·0%
For others	95·6%	91·6%	90·4%	93·4%	91·5%

Absence from school was not the cause of deterioration in the majority of cases. Here and there, however, it had its effect as an additional contributory cause. The findings of other researchers are of interest here, for example Osmend (1951), in comparing boys who were not succeeding academically at a

35

grammar school with academically successful boys, found that the former:—

(1) tended to stay away for longer periods when they were absent;
(2) were absent more frequently;
(3) showed more adverse effect in attainment after a period of absence;
(4) showed poorer estimates of character traits, especially of persistence and reliability when compared individually with successful boys who had correspondingly long spells or long duration of absence from school.

Sandon (1938) states: 'There is, in a number of secondary school pupils, a psychological or physical constitution that results in poor progress being associated with frequent absence, so much so that frequent short spells of absence are related with educational retardation more than are less frequent longer spells of much greater total duration'.

The Grammar School

The authors are well aware that the grammar school itself cannot be entirely exonerated in this enquiry into the causes of deterioration. Most of its faults, however, are not peculiar to the school of the enquiry, but common to most schools of its type. Nor do we wish to describe faults without paying tribute, even though it be in passing, to the many merits of these schools. We are, however, concerned primarily with academic deterioration and must therefore confine ourselves to its causes. We distinguish three aspects of grammar school organisation which help to produce this deterioration. The first is lack of sufficient knowledge among the staff about the home conditions of individual pupils. The second is the lack of any systematic provision for helping pupils who have, for one reason or another, fallen behind in those subjects which have a building-type of structure, like mathematics and foreign languages. The third is lack of a sufficiently close relationship between staff and children, particularly in the first year when the pupils have just come from the care of a permanent Form teacher. Because there are so many subjects taught by so many teachers, the stumbler can become nobody's business. In Chapter VI, 'Conclusions', are made various suggestions for remedying these faults.

Minor troubles

Some deteriorators travelled very long distances to school, almost always by bus. The outstanding examples of sufferers from this cause were two sisters. They walked a mile uphill every morning to exposed cross-roads and spent up to an hour in the bus to school. Five other deteriorators were similarly handicapped, but not quite as severely. Travelling by bus is particularly bad as it is difficult to do even reading homework because of the jolting, and probably injurious to attempt it for more than a few minutes.

While making the case studies we came across evidence of pupils being affected by the change from primary to secondary school. Change of school probably upsets most children, some more than others, but some also recover more quickly than others. On the whole it appeared to be the children from the smaller rural schools who were affected most. Here the change would be at its greatest—from the friendly, informal and often small 'family' class of the outbacks to the large impersonal subject-centred classes of the grammar school.

A pupils' choice of out-of-school friends sometimes had a strong effect on his or her school work. The most unfortunate associations were with children who were set little or no homework at school. There was some evidence to show that this type of association had a harmful effect on the homework of two of the girl deteriorators and eight of the boys.

Sometimes extra-mural coaching at the primary school level gains a grammar school place for pupils who would otherwise be rejected. We have, however, no information that any one of the deteriorators had received such coaching.

A Note on Subject Preference

Parents will be well aware that mathematics and foreign languages have a tendency to arouse either an intense liking or an intense dislike. Usually the liking is accompanied by good ability in the subject and dislike by poor or mediocre ability.

The attitude of the child will of course have a strong influence on his attainment. In view of this we compared the attitudes of the deteriorators with those of non-deteriorators. Though the number of deteriorators is small and the results are therefore tentative, we thought they were of sufficient interest to present as an addendum to this chapter. We found an interesting difference between the attitudes of deteriorators to mathematics and to a foreign language, compared with the attitudes of non-deteriorators. They were all asked, 'Which subject do you like least?' Of the 21 boy deteriorators 43 per cent gave mathematics and only 6.4 per cent of the group of 47 non-deteriorators. Of the 18 girl deteriorators 72.2 per cent gave mathematics, and only 25.5 per cent of a corresponding group of 55 non-deteriorating girls. The differences were statistically significant. When they were asked, 'Which is your favourite subject?' only 14 per cent of the boy deteriorators chose mathematics, but 34 per cent of the non-deteriorators, while the corresponding figures for the girls were 11 per cent and 31 per cent. For a foreign language the trends were the same but the differences were not large enough for us to be able to rely on them in view of the small number of deteriorators involved. Some confirmation of these findings is to be seen in the research of another educationist, Jones, C. V. (1962), who reported 'a statistically significant association between academic deterioration and dislike of mathematics and French'.

V

JUNIOR SCHOOL X

The Home District of School X

AS mentioned in Chapter I, Junior School X was chosen for special enquiry because it produced a higher proportion of grammar school deteriorators than did other schools. The school was situated in a district which contained some eight hundred houses. There was no social centre, apart from a few places of worship and public houses, but a town was situated a comparatively short distance from its outskirts.

About four hundred and fifty of the houses were, on the average, one hundred years old. They consisted of four (some five) small rooms, including bedrooms; they lacked modern conveniences. Their average rateable value before the revaluation was about £10. Some fifty houses were rather more substantial than those mentioned above. They were between fifty and seventy years old. There were about a hundred new Council houses, a similar number of other houses recently built, with about the same number of small bungalows.

School X

The Junior School had an average population somewhat less than 300. The average size of the class was 34·4. The classes were numbered from one to five, some with 'A' and 'B' streams.

Class 1A was the scholarship stream; Class 1B consisted of bright pupils who were too young to sit the grammar school examination plus those who were old enough to sit but very unlikely to pass. 1B was a rather large class. Five classes were in the main school building, one in a hut in the yard and two in hired rooms.

Junior School X

School X did not provide ideal conditions for teaching.[1] In spite of this there was much effective teaching in the school, as shown in the following analysis of the school scholarship examination results.

TABLE 10

Grammar School Entrance Examination

	Place Winners		Preliminary Examination	
	Girls	Boys	Girls	Boys
Year 1	10	3	No Preliminary	
Year 2	9	11	19	25
Year 3	7	10	19	22
Year 4	6	10	18	22
Year 5	6	13	21	17

The Table shows that the entry to the grammar school from School X was about 45 per cent of candidates in Year 2, over 41 per cent in Year 3, about 40 per cent in Year 4, and about 39 per cent in Year 5. The corresponding percentages for all other schools were about 38 per cent, 39 per cent, 48 per cent, 46 per cent. We see therefore that over the four years School X obtained about the same percentage of successes as the remaining schools did. This result was achieved in spite of their candidates being poorer in quality than the average. We see also from the Table below that the successful pupils must have been fairly high in the order of merit as they were placed in the higher streams in the Grammar School. (This streaming was done by order of merit).

TABLE 11

The 'streams' in which pupils from School X were placed on entrance to the Grammar School

	Girls			Boys			
Streams	A	B	C	A	B	C	(D)
Year 1	3	5	2	2	1	—	
Year 2	4	3	2	7	3	1	
Year 3	3	4	—	5	3	2	
Year 4	4	2	—	4	5	1	
Year 5	3	2	1	4	2	6	1

[1] For a discussion of the influence of junior school buildings on the success of its pupils at the entrance (to grammar school) examination, the reader is referred to Floud, op. cit, 1957.

Thirty-three girls out of 38, and 36 boys out of 47, were placed in 'A' or 'B' streams on entry into the Grammar School.

Comparison of Academic Performance of Girls and Boys from School X

Commencing in Year 2 and continuing for Years 3, 4 and 5, there occurred at the school an interesting change in the proportions of boys and girls who were successful in gaining grammar school places. A larger proportion of boys than girls entered the Grammar School from School X between Year 2 and Year 5; whereas the reverse was the case for the other schools in the area, as it had also been in School X itself. We therefore made a special examination of these four years.

TABLE 12

Grammar School entrants from School X and those from all other schools

	School X		All other schools	
	Girls	Boys	Girls	Boys
Year 2	9	11	42	28
Year 3	7	10	35	26
Year 4	6	10	42	34
Year 5	6	13	48	34
TOTAL	28	44	167	122

From the table we can see that the relative percentage entries of girls compared with boys, from all other schools (based on total entry from these schools) were 57.8 per cent and 42.2 per cent respectively; the corresponding percentage from School X (based on total entry from School X) are 38.9 per cent and 61.1 per cent[1]. This considerable percentage difference in entry between girls and boys of School X is not consistent with the relative numbers sitting the preliminary examination (q.v. Table 10) because 45 per cent of the children sitting the preliminary from School X were girls. It is unlikely that the boys of School X had greater average ability than the girls, at this age. It is interesting that Richardson (1956) states '. . . "successful" (primary) schools were much less successful

[1] The difference is statistically significant; the entry from School X for Years 2 to 5 contained a far higher proportion of boys that did the entry from all other schools combined. The overall tendency for girls to obtain a greater proportion of places is nation-wide. (Cf. Douglas, 1964, p. 74).

with girls than they were with the boys. In the grammar school, 63 per cent of the boys came from "successful" schools, but only 35 per cent of the girls'.

We then examined the amount of deterioration in the two sexes for these four years. In Table 13, for Years 2 to 5, we note that six of the girls became deteriorators (out of 28 entrants), and nine of the boys (out of 44 entrants), i.e. about a fifth of both the boys and the girls. There is no evidence here that the teacher of the boys overcoached his pupils, thus getting better results than the teacher of the girls. We must observe, however, that 11 of the 44 boys could not become 'deteriorators' according to the definition adopted, because they were already in the lowest stream, but only three of the 28 girls were so placed. When this is allowed for 24 per cent of the girls 'at risk' became deteriorators and 27.3 per cent of the boys. This difference is small and is in the same direction as in the other schools of the district. We therefore came to two conclusions. The first was that if the improvement in the proportion of boys gaining places was due to more effective teaching of the boys— or less effective teaching of the girls—these effects had not increased the proportion of deterioration. The second was that—as we had realised from the beginning—using such small numbers we could only come to dependable conclusions if we found startling differences. No such differences were found. We therefore turned to our main task, which was to compare the proportion of deteriorators from School X with the proportion from all other schools.

Comparison of the Percentage of Deteriorators from School X with that of Deteriorators from all other Primary Schools in the Area

When we compare Table 10 and Table 13, this time for all five years, we can see that there were a total of 9 girl deteriorators out of 38 entries and 10 boy deteriorators out of 47 entries, from School X, over five years; that is, 23.7 per cent of the girl entries deteriorated and 21.3 per cent of the boys. When we again consider only those 'at risk' (see Table 11) the percentages become almost identical at 27 per cent for girls and 28 per cent for boys. The deterioration from all other schools for five years, as defined in this enquiry, was 4.3 per cent for girls (9 out of 211 entries), and 6.7 per cent for boys (11 out of 165 entries). The difference *between the sexes* in academic deterioration, for pupils from all junior schools, though in the expected direction, i.e. a rather greater percentage of boys than girls (9.9 per cent against 7.2 per cent) is in this case not statistically significant.

TABLE 13

A comparison of the number of girl and boy deteriorators from School X and those from all other schools

	School X		All other schools	
	Girls	Boys	Girls	Boys
Year 1	3	1	4	3
Year 2	1	4	1	1
Year 3	2	2	1	2
Year 4	2	1	—	3
Year 5	1	2	3	2
TOTAL	9	10	9	11

Here however there is another difference, which in size is the startling difference we were looking for. No less than 22.4 per cent of the entries from School X deteriorated (19 out of 85), while only 5.3 per cent of the entries from all other schools deteriorated (20 out of 376). This 17 per cent difference in deteriorators between School X and all the other junior schools in the area is statistically highly significant. We therefore continued the search for the cause of this situation.

The Relative Influence of Junior School Teaching and Home Environment for School X and for Other Schools

From the evidence already presented we can see that School X obtained an unduly high proportion of grammar school places, if we apply as a test the success or failure of their pupils during the first year at the grammar school. The most likely reasons for such a situation are either that School X was able to drill or train a high percentage of its pupils to a higher level academically than their ability was able to maintain, or that the percentage of entrants from School X who came from 'unhelpful' homes was much higher than was the case elsewhere, and that this influence acted more powerfully when the pupil was in the grammar school than when he was in the primary school. By 'unhelpful' we mean, for example, homes where parental opinion did not support school work, or where there was lack of facilities for study. In order to clarify the matter a more detailed comparison was made between the deteriorators from School X and those from other schools. Each case study was taken individually, and examined carefully for the 'principal factor' behind the deterioration. In many cases there appeared to be little doubt about this, but wherever there seemed to be some doubt the decision was made by the co-author who did not know whether the pupil came from School X or not. Though the final allocation was inevitably subjective, a determined attempt was made to remove any possible bias.

The case studies are classified in Tables 14 and 15 according to principal factors only, in so far as they could be identified, under four headings. One pupil has not been included as we were unable in his case to select a principal factor. There were also a few cases where there was a contributory factor which was almost as powerful as the principal one. Classification of this kind is difficult, and the table must therefore be regarded as somewhat tentative, in spite of the exhaustive examination which we gave jointly to each case.

Although the overall numbers are admittedly small for this type of work it must be remembered that each case is a severe example of academic deterioration, collected together over five years, and selected objectively. We consider, therefore that the general trends of the comparison between pupils from School X and those from other schools should be reasonably reliable.

The heading 'Personal Factors' has lack of persistence (in the pupil himself) as its main constituent. 'Emotional Upsets' embraces two cases where the pupil experienced severe emotional crises which, though originally in the home, were not due to a poor home background. The 'Lack of Ability' section does not of course include pupils who were placed in the bottom stream on entrance. The percentages are included only to aid the reader to perceive at a glance the general character of the results and are not intended to be read as precise figures. Those percentages based on one or two cases only must inevitably be very imprecise and unreliable, and they are given only to complete the 100 per cent.

TABLE 14

Principal Factors in the Deterioration of each pupil[1]

| | School X | | Other Schools | |
	Girls	Boys	Girls	Boys
Lack of intellectual ability	1(11%)	1(11%)	0	0
Unsupporting home background	6(67%)	5(56%)	8(89%)	6(55%)
Personal factors	2(22%)	3(33%)	0	4(36%)
Emotional upsets	0	0	1(11%)	1(9%)
TOTALS	9(100%)	9(100%)	9(100%)	11(100%)

Table 14 is based on only thirty-eight cases; but it gives once again an indication that home background is an important factor in deterioration. We should perhaps repeat that there is more than one cause of deterioration in many cases; an attempt has been made here to find the main cause for each pupil. In the above table, however, where the analysis examines the relative proportions of the principal causes *within each group of deteriorators*, there are no reliable differences.

If we use the evidence in a different way, the chief factor producing the difference between School X and the other schools is shown. In the table below the incidence of the cause of deterioration is percentaged against the total number of entrants from that particular school or group of schools. The table is deliberately confined to three of the factors, namely lack of intellectual ability, unsupporting home background, and personal factors.

TABLE 15

Deteriorators, Percentaged Against Relevant Entrants

| | School X | | Other Schools | |
	Girls	Boys	Girls	Boys
Lack of intellectual ability	1 (2·6%)	1 (2·1%)	0	0
Unsupporting home background	6 (15·8%)	5 (10·6%)	8 (3·8%)	6 (3·6%)
Personal factors	2 (5·3%)	3 (6·4%)	0	4 (2·4%)
Total Entrants	38	47	211	165

The number of cases is too small for any reliance to be

[1] The percentages are included as a rough guide.

45

placed on the difference between the schools under 'Lack of intellectual ability'. On the other hand the differences between the schools under the heading 'Unsupporting home background' are too large to be ignored and are statistically highly significant[1]. The influence of a poor home background is much more widespread in the catchment area of School X when compared with the catchment areas of all other primary schools. When one takes a walk in the neighbourhood this becomes abundantly clear. The influence of the neighbourhood itself, particularly its social and education outlook, appeared to us to be very powerful, but our work did not include any attempt to isolate it from the influence of the home.

Since analysis of the causes of deterioration in the academic progress of entrants from School X seemed to point to the character of the homes as a major factor in the deterioration, it was decided to make a more detailed enquiry into the home background of the deteriorators from School X. The home of each deteriorator was visited at least once; in some cases more than one visit was necessary to check on previous impressions.

An indication of the social status of a community can be obtained from a knowledge of the types of occupation pursued by its members. An investigation of parental occupation, therefore, was carried out in the School X district; the categories into which the occupations are divided were based on the 'Standard Classification for Social Status of Occupation' (Glass, 1954). The categories are outlined in Chapter I. The result of the investigation is shown in Table 16.

The table shows that School X district contained a preponderance of parents in semi-skilled occupation; there was, also, nearly twice the percentage of unskilled workers in the district compared to all primary school districts in the area of the grammar school. It is significant that there was only one resident in School X district marked 'J' (for Juror) on the electoral roll.

The evidence therefore points strongly to the following analysis. School X is situated in a district which is materially and culturally much less advanced than the average standard

---

[1] The Chi-square test: significant beyond the ·oo1 level, when the 2×2 table contrasts pupils with a poor home background with 'all others' and School X with all other schools.

of the other districts which feed the grammar school. By either exceptionally good teaching or maybe special coaching, and certainly by hard work on the part of both staff and pupils, School X gained a much higher proportion of grammar school places than would normally have been expected from a school situated in such an area. When these pupils reached the grammar school, however, the differential teaching effect which brought many of them there was removed, and some

TABLE 16

Social Status from Parental Occupation

Category of Parental Occupation	1	2	3	4	5	6	7
School X District (Years 1 to 5)	—	—	1%	2%	22%	65%	10%
All other School Districts (Year 5)	5·9%	8·8%	9·8%	8·8%	40·2%	20·6%	5·9%

Category 5 indicates skilled manual and routine grades of non-manual etc.; Category 6 indicates semi-skilled labour; Category 7 indicates unskilled.

'deterioration' would naturally occur. This process would be exacerbated by the probably greater influence of the homes on progress in the grammar school than on progress in the primary school. As we are not here concerned with those pupils who just scraped in to the grammar school, and who were therefore placed in the bottom stream, the main cause of deterioration is not lack of ability, but inadequate motivation for academic work, stemming often from a home background which gave inadequate support, but finding its roots in the ethos of the neighbourhood. The relatively low standard of parental education in such a district is only one of many factors which impinge on the problem, and it is closely related to a number of others. This study, however, shows dramatically its importance.

Improvers from School X

Late in this work we thought that an examination of the few 'improvers' from the same school might throw into relief the salient factors accounting for the decline of the deteriorators. In Years 1 and 2 there were no improvers among the boys from School X, but three of the 19 girl entrants (16%) showed substantial improvement. Taking entrants from all other junior schools in the grammar school area for the same period, improvement was shown by five of the 86 girl entrants (6%) and two of the 71 boys entrants (3%).

If the matter had been left there readers would have been given a misleading impression, because during the next four years there was no other improver, either boy or girl, from this school, although there were 26 from other primary schools.

The three girl improvers from School X did not, as one might have expected, have parents who were educated in a grammar school. This would indeed have been exceptional in this district. They all belonged, however to social class 5, which except for 3 per cent of parents, was the highest class of the district. They also lived in houses which were appreciably better than most of the houses in the catchment area. They were all the first-born members of the family, and in two of the cases there were only two children in the family. Most important of all was the supporting nature of the parental attitude to the children's education, evidenced in a number of ways (Cf. Whalley (1961) p. 142). All three girls also showed a good standard of persistence during their school careers. This undoubtedly originated partly in the parental attitude, but there may also have been a contribution from the inherited temperamental characteristics of the girls. Their ability, however, was limited and none of them set the Thames on fire in their external examinations.

As in the case of deterioration, the sex difference in the incidence of academic 'improvement' is in favour of the girls, i.e. there is a greater proportion of boy deteriorators and of girl improvers among the grammar school entrants who came from School X. The numbers are so small that we checked the trend by comparing it with the overall results for Years 1 to 5. As indicated at the beginning of this chapter, there were 9.9 per cent of deteriorators amongst the boys and 7.2 per cent among the girls. On the other hand there were 7.2 per cent of improvers among the girls and only 4.7 per cent among the boys. The trend is slight, but it agrees with the findings of other research. (Cf. Rushton (1963), pp. 3 and 117).

VI

CONCLUSIONS

THIS survey was made in one grammar school only and its findings are based on a relatively small number of pupils. It was a clinical study designed to explore in detail the reasons underlying the deterioration which has been exposed by statistical studies, and as it had only one part-time field worker, this limitation in breadth was inevitable. We cannot, therefore, say that we have proved that our findings are applicable to all secondary grammar schools in England and Wales, and though we ourselves can see no reason why the general tenor of them should not be applicable to other secondary schools, we would welcome the appearance of other detailed studies investigating the same problems. Other research has indeed already pointed in the same general direction as this work. Apart from well known published sources there is much evidence buried in recent research theses such as those of Whalley (1961) and Rushton (1963).

This survey has examined, in particular, academic deterioration in the first year of attendance, when the highest percentage of deterioration usually occurs (cf. Valentine, 1932, pp. 84–5). The authors considered that this was the most important stage for diagnosis, when pupils were endeavouring to adjust themselves to the new environment. In addition, research shows that the rank order at the end of the first year agrees more closely with results in the General Certificate of Education than does the rank order in the entrance examination. (Cf. Whalley, 1961, pp. 98–9). For this and other reasons our deteriorators and improvers do not include pupils who commenced their deterioration or improvement after their first year in the grammar school. All the 39 deteriorators and the 36 improvers selected themselves by the end of their first year.

There are many causes of academic deterioration. They may begin at the very birth of the child, yet be quiescent for years. They may start at any time, and cease as suddenly; but it is easier for them to start than for their effects to disappear. Junior and grammar school, home and neighbourhood, friends and enemies, all contribute their quota, and even John and Margaret themselves, the deteriorators in the flesh, may sometimes be held responsible. Society is the setting for this little drama, and society often has its effect on the outcome of the play. Some causes are mainly intellectual, others fundamentally emotional, and it is perhaps surprising that in a grammar school where there is a large percentage entry, but where the standard of attainment demanded must be fairly high, the chief cause of deterioration is to be found in the attitude of the pupil and not in his level of ability, though the causes of his attitude are many and varied.

In order to succeed at a grammar school a pupil must have at least average academic aptitude and a willingness to work. If the aptitude is at the minimum level the persistence must be great, whereas if the aptitude is high there is not the same need for intense application to studies. In only two cases out of the 39 deteriorators did we find that lack of intellectual ability was the main cause of deterioration, though in several other cases it was a contributory factor. Using the evidence in another way, we found only two cases in a five-year entry comprising 461 pupils. At first sight this again may seem very surprising, particularly for a school which admits more than 40 per cent of the relevant age group each year. If we think a little more deeply, however, the finding becomes more understandable. The level of aptitude demanded during the first year is merely that which, combined with persistence, will enable pupils to compete adequately with their fellow-entrants. In other words, the standard demanded will tend to be relative rather than absolute. It follows that only very good teaching, or possibly cramming (or maybe a mistake), can secure grammar school entrance for a pupil of inadequate academic aptitude. Now most pupils who secure entrance in this manner will appear in the bottom third of the order of merit and be allocated to the lowest stream, and by our self-imposed definition of deterioration we are not concerned with those who enter in this stream. In addition, the difference in the teaching efficiency of junior school teachers taking the 'scholarship class', where there is a high and common motivation for both teachers and taught, is unlikely to be so great as to cause of itself a dramatic decline in the order of merit of many pupils in the grammar school, when this Junior school differential has been removed. Readers will remember that those pupils who deteriorated merely from the 'A' to the 'B' stream have not been classed as deteriorators.

Further evidence on this point is provided by a comparison which we made of the average I.Q. of ten 'deteriorators' and ten 'improvers' from School X. The former scored an average I.Q. of 113 and the latter scored 110. Again, when we compared the I.Q. of all the deteriorators from a two-year entry with that of other pupils of the same sex who were paired with them for place in the entrance examination, the average I.Q. of the deteriorators was 112.9, and that of the 'control' pupils 110.2. The average I.Q. of all the 39 deteriorators was 111.4, with a range of about 124 to 100. The rank order of the deteriorators (Year 5) on entrance provides an additional pointer. When we compared them with the improvers for that year we found that, except for one improver, all the deteriorators gained a higher rank order on entrance. This was, of course, almost pre-determined by the definitions adopted; deteriorators, in order to be designated as such, could not be in a really low position on entrance, and vice versa for improvers.

With regard to pupil attainment, of particular interest were the elementary faults in the mechanical processes of Arithmetic which were exposed by the Schonell Diagnostic Arithmetic Test. That one pupil should consistently multiply wrongly by nought, that two others should similarly omit 'internal' noughts in the answer to a division sum, that two others should fail to understand the basic principles of multiplication by double figures—to give only a few examples—is a situation which ought not to exist with pupils whose intelligence is average or above. The periodic administration of scientifically designed diagnostic tests of arithmetic and a remedial follow-up to correct the specific misunderstandings of individuals should be a *sine qua non* of good teaching—where classes are not too large and the money is available. Even these difficulties might be overcome. Nor should this process of scientific testing end with the junior school. It may be that teaching machines, provided with the precise programme for eradicating the fault, would have a part to play here. Neglect of such faults would cause first bewilderment and low attainment, and later an emotional resistance to the subject which might even spread to include school in general.

As lack of academic aptitude was not a major cause of deterioration we come to the second cause, the attitude of the pupil to work. The difference between those pupils who made normal progress (or improved) and those who deteriorated was largely determined by the nature of their application to academic work. In its turn this was decided by the interaction of the innate persistence of the pupil with his emotional attitude to this work, which was strongly influenced by his home background.

Before examining the forces affecting the pupils' attitude we shall first take a particular aspect of the attitude of our deteriorators which seems important; this is their attitude to Mathematics. Whereas 72 per cent of the girl deteriorators disliked Mathematics more than any other subject, only 25 per cent of girls making normal progress disliked the subject more than any other; the figures for the boys were 43 per cent and 6 per cent. The differences for both sexes between deteriorators and 'normals' are statistically highly significant and though our numbers are small the results are supported by similar findings in the work of C. V. Jones (1962). The same finding may well be true with regard to Modern Languages (supported also by C. V. Jones). In the present survey, however, the differences in the latter, though in the expected direction, were not statistically significant, perhaps because pupils could choose one out of three languages.

The attitude of pupils to their studies can be affected by a great variety of influences. Some of these influences are sudden and dramatic, others insidious and persistent; the extent to which they affect work is largely decided by the character of the boy and the nature of his home background. In a very few cases we decided that the pupil himself or herself was mainly at fault, through his or her neglect of homework. In these cases the home background in general was good, though the lack of a sufficiently firm home discipline was sometimes a minor contributory factor in the decline. The pupils so classified were much more interested in other activities than in bookwork at home—usually girls in social engagements (one girl deteriorator was sexually precocious), and boys in sports. In one case only did we ascribe the neglect to an unbalanced temperament, a view which was confirmed by later events.

In most of the cases of deterioration it was the nature of the home which was the decisive force in moulding the attitude of the pupil. In a few instances the deteriorator was emotionally disturbed by some aspect of home life that could not be changed. It is not easy, for instance, to recover from the shock of suddenly discovering that you are illegitimate. In another case deterioration appeared to be due to the death of a mother, and in yet another the serious prolonged illness of a parent seemed to be a strong contributory factor.

In contrast to the relatively small incidence of these 'acts of God' there were many other aspects of the home background which adversely affected the progress of most of the deteriorators. These aspects ranged from the lack of proper facilities for doing homework, through a parental *laissez-faire* attitude to discipline, to severe emotional disharmony in the home. Of all these aspects undoubtedly emotional disharmony was the most disturbing to the child, and the most harmful to satisfactory progress in school work. In no less than one quarter of the cases there was strong evidence of this factor. At this stage in the analysis we appear to have a paradox. The research has demonstrated the strong relationship between deterioration and social class and between deterioration and the type of education of the parents. No deteriorator had a parent who was placed higher than category 4 for social class. Does this mean that there was no serious disharmony in the homes of pupils belonging to classes above category 4? This is scarcely credible, but how otherwise can the discrepancy be explained? The authors make no claim to have solved this problem but suggest the following hypothesis.

It may be that the type of conduct which results from disharmony in the home belonging to social categories 1 to 3

Conclusions

(and maybe 4) is of a kind which produces much less emotional stress in the child than does the type of conduct customary among categories 5 to 7. For example, the husbands belonging to categories 1 to 3 are much less likely to have recourse to physical assault on their wives, whether drunk or sober, than the husbands belonging to categories 5 to 7. It may be also that it is usual for the husbands and wives of the 'upper' and 'middle' classes to avoid inflicting their more serious disputes on their children, while among the 'lower' classes this is not so. Again, the child who experiences serious disharmony in the home will be driven to look for some refuge or some activity outside it. The 'upper class' child will have recourse to relatives and friends of the same class and, of the same outlook on education, and thus will be supported in his studies; the 'lower' class child will also look for support to relatives and friends of his own social class, but these will not tend to have as strong a supporting attitude to education, and deterioration may set in.

This survey shows that social class factors were undoubtedly associated with deterioration in a large majority of the 39 cases. Whereas the 36 improvers came from social classes 2 to 5, all but two of the 39 deteriorators came from classes 5 to 7. The two exceptions came from class 4. Of pupils whose fathers were in the unskilled category, about one third of the five-year entry became deteriorators (10 out of 30). Of those with semi-skilled fathers slightly more than a tenth became deteriorators (12 out of 110). In the skilled category the percentage was approximately 8 (15 out of 194). There was no deterioration, as defined, among the children of the higher social classes, but there were improvers. None of these improvers had fathers who belonged to a social class category below 5, i.e. that of the skilled manual worker. These findings are very similar to those of Whalley (1961), and other researchers.

Related to the social class of the parent is the type of education they themselves received. One of the most startling findings of this research is that *only one parent out of more than seventy belonging to the deteriorators had been educated in a grammar school.* On the other hand we must point out that there were six improvers out of 36 whose parents had not attended a grammar school; these, however, were exceptions to the general rule. In contrast to the finding for deteriorators we discovered that in a

E   55

normal 2-year entry 108 families out of 181 had one or more parents educated at a grammar school. We have already seen that when this 2-year entry was itself classified according to its streaming and the parental education it was found that only 15 per cent of the children who had no parent educated in a grammar school were in the 'A' stream, while 53 per cent were in the 'C' stream. When both parents had attended a grammar school 62 per cent of the children were in the 'A' stream and only 6 per cent in the 'C' stream. Unfortunately we were unable, from the data at our disposal, to separate out the parental education factor from the father's social class.

What factors connected with social class, other than parental education, are responsible for this strong effect upon pupil attainment? In this age of the Welfare State there must be many who have said that poverty could not possibly be a force of any importance. They would be wrong. Much depends on what is meant by poverty. It is true that the stark poverty of Edwardian times—or maybe of the thirties—when children went barefoot, wore rags and were obviously under-nourished, has largely gone. Still with us, however, are the small mean houses, with far too few rooms for the number of occupants. With us too are many homes where the family income, though sufficient to pay for a fire in the living-room, is inadequate for a second fire in a separate room where homework could be done without interruption. We have seen that in no fewer than 20 cases of deterioration, out of the 39, there was evidence of the lack of a fire in any room other than the kitchen or living-room. And the room with the fire would be the room with the television set or radio.

Poverty—or financial stringency—also exerts its influence in ways other than material. Attitudes are more important than facilities, and financial stringency can certainly have a powerful effect on the former. Though we have definite knowledge of only two cases where children were told that they would be withdrawn from school at the first opportunity, with a resultant lack of incentive in their schoolwork, there may well have been others who were affected in the same way. We discovered five cases in all where poverty was a strong factor in the pupils' deterioration.

A closely related, but not identical factor, is the size of

family. In the preceding chapter we illustrated the strong relationship between the size of family and the academic performance of the children. Though the numbers in our comparison of the family size of deteriorators and improvers were too small for statistical verification, this effect persisted within each social class in which both types of case were present. As the size of the family increased so the attainment of the pupils tended to fall. Nor is this to be wondered at, since eleven of our deteriorators, when doing homework, experienced constant interruption from other members of the family—mainly younger children. Parents of large families are also often too busy looking after the younger children, or too tired, to be able to give much attention to the children's homework, whereas the parents of a small family have more time and energy to devote to each child. Hence we see that 24 out of the 36 improvers were the first-born, and apart from the one exceptional case of a professional man's family only two of these families had as many as four children, twenty-six of the families having only two or less.

Another important aspect of the home, for our purpose, is its level of culture. The child from the upper and middle social classes has a flying start over his working class rivals in richness of vocabulary and in general knowledge. The conversation of the parents will be more informative, he will visit more places and have readier access to a wide variety of books. The first-born in any family will benefit in a somewhat similar way as he will tend to converse frequently with his parents, whereas children born later in the family will tend to talk much more to their brothers and sisters. Children from the upper and middle classes and also first-born children will, in addition, tend to receive more parental tutoring when they are doing their homework. This can be a great boon to children who have been absent from school, and have missed 'key' lessons in subjects such as Mathematics and Modern Language, where the learning of a new step often depends upon the understanding of a previous one.

In the preceding paragraphs on poverty and on the size of the family we have touched on the attitude of the parents towards the child's studies. This factor, however, deserves a section to itself because a favourable attitude is crucial for the

E*   57

child's success. Often, of course, this effect may be seen in reverse, the success of the child creating a favourable attitude in the parent. More pertinent to this study is the failure of the child creating a parental attitude of despondency or an attitude which results in the withdrawal of positive support. This feed-back effect, which lurks in the background of studies of this nature, and is occasionally not detected, was at its minimum in this study. This is because the period under review was the child's first year in the grammar school, immediately after the success of the child in gaining a place. Attitudes are rarely changed overnight, and it would take some months for the parental joy in their offspring's achievement to become at first surprise and then despair.

Attitudes produced by severe emotional disharmony between the parents or between parent and child can have a catastrophic effect on a pupil's attainment. Less obvious, but also important is the effect of the day by day commentary by the parents on the school, on homework and on books. Other pointers to the parental attitude are the priority they give to homework over other activities, the frequency of constructive interviews with the Headmaster, attendance at school functions, and extent to which the casual absences of the child from school are with their tacit consent or active connivance. Slowly but surely the parental comments and their scale of priorities have their effect on the attitude of the child. Even a parental attitude of neutrality or *laissez-faire* is a big handicap to a child who is competing against other children who have fully supporting parents.

In this study we have found that the pupils with unsupporting home backgrounds who become deteriorators tended to come from social classes 5, 6 and 7, while the improvers came from social classes 2, 3, 4 and 5 and most of them had good supporting backgrounds. The child of a professional man will usually get far better support at home for his studies than the child of an unskilled labourer. This does not deny that there are exceptions to the general rule, but the average tendencies are more informative to us than are the exceptions.

This summary of the effect of the home background would not be complete without some consideration of the influence of the neighbourhood on the attitude of both parents and pupils to academic work. The story that is told of a labourer who came home, saw his boy doing his homework and swept the books off the table, shouting 'What you doin' that bloody stuff for?' may or may not be true, and this attitude is now passing, but in a much milder form it typifies the attitude of some neighbourhoods. More usually the expressed attitude is merely neutral rather than positive. But the pupils' friends have their evenings free and are playing football or cricket or going to the cinema while our deteriorator should be doing his homework. In these districts the accepted and expected leaving age is fifteen, while in higher class neighbourhoods it is eighteen, or increasingly, twenty-two or more. Our analysis, however, did not extend to the making of an assessment of the prevalent attitudes to grammar school education in the various districts of the catchment area. To conclude this section we feel it necessary to say outright, in case we are misunderstood, that it is by no means the intention of the authors to disparage the manual working classes, or to praise the professional and executive classes. We detest snobbery as much as anyone and are ourselves of working class and lower middle class origins. Rather do we wish to analyse the situation as objectively as we can, in order to discover where there are weaknesses and to suggest possible remedies.

While we consider that the character of the home background exerted a powerful influence on academic progress in the grammar school we cannot dismiss lightly the possibility that inherited personality characteristics, correlated to some extent with social class, may also have been at work. Though the evidence points away from lack of intelligence as a factor in producing the deteriorators, it is possible that a social class difference in temperamental tendencies—partly inherited— may have been partly responsible. One of the most important of these characteristics would be persistence. For example, some families may belong to the 'unskilled labourer' class primarily because of the fathers' lack of persistence. Those temperamental traits which lead to the development of such a character may well be inherited by some children, though they are acquired by others through imitation. On this point we have little evidence, as lack of resources prevented us from establishing a control group of case studies of pupils who had made normal progress, against which we could have evaluated the case studies of deteriorators. Whatever their origin there do appear to be differences between the social classes in temperamental outlook and conduct in the school situation. Halsey and Gardner (1953) found, for example, that for 13 to 14 year old boys in grammar schools those of middle class origin have, on the whole, higher ratings for industriousness, sense of responsibility, interest in school affairs, good behaviour and good manners. Nor is it likely that these differences are attributable mainly to the middle-class outlook of the raters.

Other minor causes of deterioration, such as absence from school, failure to wear spectacles, undetected deafness, we shall pass over quickly, because although they were important in a few individual cases, they do not rank as major causes. But before we pass on to a consideration of remedial measures there is one aspect of the problem which should be put before readers.

This aspect is the nature of the transition from primary to secondary school. At the former the pupil stays in one room for most of the day and is taught by one teacher. This teacher sees the same pupils for most of the day and for five days a week. He therefore acquires a thorough knowledge of each pupil's temperament and ability. In the scholarship class, especially, it is not easy for a child to be slack; he is made to work, nor can his home background do much to interfere actively with his progress. When, however, the child enters the grammar school he comes, at a tender age, to a quite different environment, where his teachers change from lesson to lesson in a kaleidoscopic fashion, where he is plunged into many strange subjects, and where he is no longer one of the oldest but one of the youngest in the school. His uniform is new, his pals are gone. No longer is the school just round the corner—it may be an hour's journey, in all kinds of weather. Above all, whereas previously the teacher preparing him for the 11 plus examination had provided him with the necessary persistence, now he is left much more to paddle his own canoe. Gone is the very close supervision of the primary school—and some pupils are unable to substitute their own persistence.

Having surveyed the causes of deterioration, we now come to the remedies.

In the grammar school the problem of deterioration centres upon the attitude of the child to academic work. In so far as our school buildings are dull, depressing places they will *ipso facto* depress his interest in his work. In so far as his teachers are dull and uninspired they will affect him in the same way, but more sharply. In so far as his curriculum is traditional and uninteresting, will he tend to leave early, unenlightened and maybe even hostile. In so far as his school buildings are gracious, his teachers enthusiastic and absorbing, his curriculum up to date, his level of response will tend to be raised.

No grammar school can escape all responsibility for the failures within its doors. To some children, it is true, the school can give little help; the source of their trouble lies elsewhere, as we have seen in this study. In a few cases the school will be directly responsible, through those imperfections of character to which even the teaching profession, like other mortals, is prone. We are not here concerned with this very small percentage of cases. There are, however, several reforms in grammar schools that we believe would be helpful.

One of the most important of these is a reduction in the size of classes. It has been suggested once or twice before, but put on one side as impracticable. For impracticable read too expensive. If the pillars of the Establishment were compelled to send their own children to maintained grammar or comprehensive schools, the reform would be quickly effected. Many of the married women teachers who are not practising their profession would be tempted out of their fortresses by various devices such as much higher Income Tax allowances, and those authorities who are refusing to appoint married women could be firmly told where their duty lies. Strange though it may seem, the prospect of smaller classes would in itself be an encouragement to married teachers to flock to the rescue. This reform is more far-reaching than appears on the surface. It is not suggested as an attempt to raise the general standard of attainment, because research has yet to show that the standard does rise as the numbers in the class fall. (Though some research has purported to show that the opposite takes place, one fears that due account has not been taken of the tendency for Heads to make the dull streams and backward classes deliberately small. Besides, what Head in his senses would give an outsize class to a poor teacher if he could possibly avoid doing so?) Rather is the purpose to make the teaching more individual, with the double objective of suiting it to the individual's needs and of enabling the teacher to get to know the pupils better. The reform would incidentally help the teacher to look after such mundane but important things as the detection of weak sight and poor hearing, the wearing of spectacles, the child with enlarged adenoids, etc. Various advantages also accrue to the teacher; the strain in the classroom is reduced and the burden of marking is not as great. Both should help him to preserve the freshness of his teaching over a longer period. The suggestion is, however, made primarily because both this enquiry and the writers' long and varied teaching experience have convinced them that if the attitudes of deteriorators are to be changed their teachers need to have a better understanding of the difficulties the children may be facing. The writers themselves confess that their own knowledge of their pupils did not equip them to do this job adequately.

Another method of 'getting to know Johnnie' is the old institution of Form Masters. Most grammar schools have a master responsible for each Form, but organisational difficulties sometimes make the system less effective than it should be. Pupils in their first year should, however, have a Form Master who takes them preferably for several subjects, or alternatively for a subject which the form takes at least once a day. This should help the school to acquire a better knowledge of the newly arrived pupils, and also help the pupils to acquire a sense of 'belonging'. Of course, many schools already use this method. What is needed also, however, is a briefing from the Head to the form teacher about any 'special cases' when they enter the school, and a well maintained liaison afterwards. This often appears to be neglected.

Parent-Teacher Associations, and Open Days, etc. are other ways of getting a more useful knowledge of the children's problems. Though these associations have not been popular in some areas they should be more feasible now that the attitude towards education has so much improved. In the United States these associations donate large sums for special purposes to their local school and take a very great interest in its activities. There is no reason why such an attitude should not gradually develop over here; in fact it is already in existence in many boarding and a few day schools.

There is nothing in the least revolutionary in the above suggestions. This is not as true about some which follow. Since the principal factor which appears to affect the pupils' attitude to their work is the home background, it is with this that we should mostly concern ourselves. Any proposal that we should pry into the Englishman's castle would rightly be viewed with alarm, and the problem must be approached with circumspection. One should offer help rather than criticism, and wherever possible seek to give this help in general rather than to individuals whose carefully hidden problems have been ruthlessly exposed. The next question is the setting up of the necessary administrative machinery.

Though the Head of a school will always quite rightly have much to do with educational guidance, the problem is now too big for him to tackle alone, and it is also becoming too specialised. We need in each large grammar or comprehensive school a full-time Educational Guidance Tutor. He should be an experienced teacher, usually a graduate, with also qualifications in psychology. He would be required to work under the guidance of the Head and in close co-operation with the staff. His job would include guidance in the selection of alternative subjects, educational advice on careers, remedial teaching with individuals or small groups of juniors, and a close investigation of cases of academic deterioration or of abnormal disciplinary trouble. It is with academic deterioration that we are particularly concerned. Here the trail will often lead to the home, and the Tutor should have the services of a local authority Social Case Worker who would be attached to a small group of schools[1]. She would replace the present Welfare Officer. It would be her duty, when requested by the Tutor, to visit the deteriorator's home to talk over the matter with the parents. The Tutor's part of this work would be to give any special tests that were needed, to interview the boy, and to present the collated information at a meeting with the Head and the Social Case Worker. The staff should also be given all the information

[1] Since this was written the Newsom Report has made the same recommendation (para. 204). Cf. also para. 233 on vocational guidance.

which is not strictly confidential. Such a system would ensure that the problem cases had prompt and skilled attention.

In smaller schools the Educational Guidance Tutor would teach for a proportion of his time—probably not more than half, and the Social Case Worker would serve a larger number of schools. Such an Educational Guidance Tutor would not be a graduate in psychology, but in addition to the normal teaching qualifications he should have followed a special course of training for a year, in a University. The work of these less highly trained Tutors should be assisted by a local authority Educational Guidance Officer who would be a psychologist who had special training for this work.

Many homes and many struggling pupils would also be helped if local authorities provided rooms in which pupils could do homework under supervision. In Bootle this provision has been in existence in a library building for some years and the Librarian reports 'Greater use had been made of the Study room by children both for individual homework and for school project studies'.[1] It is probably in the towns that the need is greatest and can be met most easily. The system used in Bootle has the added advantage of bringing pupils to the library who might not otherwise be introduced to it.

The provision of facilities for doing homework is something, but it is not enough. Nor is it enough if we also give the pupil the right attitude to his work. Much of his effort must be spent in the learning of facts. But this learning requires certain techniques, and it is nobody's business to teach these techniques or even mention them. Does the child of eleven, straight from the primary school and new to homework, know the best way to work at the chapter in the text-book which he has been set to read for homework? Does he know the importance of attempting to recall what he has read, the importance of compiling and memorising a simple framework, so that the chapter becomes a meaningful entity? Does he know the technique of overlearning poetry or, with suitable poems, of learning the whole instead of the bits? Some pupils do, but some don't, and it should no longer be left to chance, but made the specific responsibility—with a few kindred topics—of the Form Masters of Forms I.

[1] County Borough of Bootle. Libraries, Annual Report, 1962-3, p. 8.

Finally we would urge that all schools should allocate provision for remedial teaching in their timetables, for those subjects such as mathematics and foreign languages in which the knowledge is built up, as it were, brick upon brick, with the solidity of the structure depending upon the solidity of the earlier work. At the moment this remedial work is left too much to chance—to the attention of an already over-worked mathematics teacher, the doubtful help of a parent, or the tenacity and determination of the individual pupil. These remedial classes would take place when there were no normal classes in this type of subject. It is envisaged that these classes would not be merely for 'backward pupils', but for pupils who were referred to it for investigation of special difficulties, for getting up-to-date after absence, etc. Such systematisation and scientific approach to remedial work appears to be badly needed, and at the same time not too difficult to put into practice.

Let it be said immediately that just as perfection is not of this world, so the phenomenon of deterioration will always be with us. Homes cannot be standardised, attitudes turned out to a common pattern, families restricted by edict to an optimum size. The untimely death of a parent, severe prolonged illness and illegitimacy, are not in our power to control. Drink may ruin a father, weak discipline spoil a child. We can do little, if anything, to alter these things. We can only ameliorate—never produce a Utopia. Indeed, if we did achieve perfection the world would probably be a very dull place. None the less there is still room for improvement before the drive towards perfection threatens us with monotony.

Reforms may improve the general standard of grammar school entrants but, strange as it may seem, these will do little or nothing to reduce the number of deteriorators. If all pupils increased their level of attainment, some would still be at the top and others at the bottom. Our examination system is essentially based on the principle of comparison between those examined. If some go up in order of merit, others must come down. If some pass in the General Certificate of Education, others must fail. Indeed if there were no failures for several years the incentive to work hard would partly be removed. The only way of escape from this situation is by replacement of the subjective and relative type of standard by a fixed standard.

This could be done by a controlled and limited use of objective tests. If these were used in conjunction with the more usual type of academic examination there would be little risk of the tests dominating the curriculum, and we would acquire a yardstick by which progress could be measured.

A reform which would take cognisance of the powerful social class forces about which much of this book has been concerned would be a relaxing of the rigidity of the tripartite system of secondary education. Since we cannot with justice allow for social class influences by excluding from the grammar schools those children who have 'unsupporting' homes, nor with justice exclude those pupils with 'supporting' homes who are just below the acceptance line, but would probably be successful there, we must seek another remedy. Fortunately such a remedy—the movement towards greater elasticity, has now been in existence for some time and is likely to increase in momentum. It will not produce the millenium, but it will bring us much nearer to a just system of allocation to secondary education. At the same time the emerging and fortunately peaceful social revolution is raising academic standards and rapidly improving the national attitude towards education. With this improvement in attitude the differential effects of the social class forces affecting children's academic performance will gradually be reduced, and the focus of the problem will tend to move towards the individual home.

The improvement in the attitude of the working classes towards education would be expedited by reforms in the curriculum of the grammar school itself. A working class boy who attends a grammar school is caught in a 'culture conflict' situation. The very middle-class outlook of the grammar school demands conformity during schooldays, while at other times the pupil is claimed by the realistic, down-to-earth and practical world of his family, friends and neighbourhood. The grammar school should seek consciously to reduce this clash of cultures, not by any debasing of its own standards but by acknowledging the problem and devising ways to meet it. One method would be to make adequate provision for practical and technical activities; these the working classes understand and respect. Any reader who maintains that we do this already should take a trip to the United States to have his eyes opened.

There, in many a high school, he will see large 'halls' full of different kinds of machinery; when compared with our own schools it is like seeing a vision from the future. These are, of course 'comprehensive' schools in organisation, but the practical and technical education which is provided is the type which should be available to pupils in our grammar schools— and is particularly suitable for many working-class children. Nor would the author seek to reduce the standards of academic excellence which the grammar schools have already achieved. This widening of provision should improve the attitude of the working-class community towards the schools, affect the attitude of the working-class children and ultimately result in a rise of academic standards rather than a fall. *Reculer pour mieux sauter.*

VII

SELECTED CASE STUDIES: DETERIORATORS, IMPROVERS

IN visiting the homes, it had to be remembered that formality would be out of place. No record of replies to questions was made at the home itself, and the caller was careful to avoid giving the impression that he was paying an official visit as a representative of the grammar school. Information was sought however, under the following headings, and an attempt was made to secure as much objective data as possible. Though all such data has been used in the investigation, it has been necessary to suppress some facts here and there to preserve the anonymity of the pupils. The headings used were:—

(a) the attitude of parents to the junior and grammar schools,
(b) the education of the parents,
(c) size of family; position of the pupil in the family,
(d) relationship between members of the family,
(e) poverty or wealth; size and character of house and number of people per room,
(f) accommodation for doing homework, e.g., whether separate room with fire.
(h) encouragement in the form of books in the home; titles of newspapers and magazines,
(i) out-of-school friendships of the children,
(j) leisure time activities and hobbies of the children.

What could not be gathered objectively was gleaned subjectively. It should be pointed out that since evidence from the homes was partly subjective, there might have been a tendency to brand a home as bad because its children were

68

deteriorators. Awareness of this bias, and the incorporation of many objective measures reduced the danger of committing the error. Sixteen of the 39 case studies of deterioration are given here, and, for contrast, case studies of four of the ten improvers for whom case studies were made.

In passing we give a few illuminating details about the later careers of a few of the deteriorators, whose problems and difficult conduct by no means ended when they left school. One youth joined an Army Apprentice School, was dismissed for indiscipline and later appeared in court for threatening with a flick-knife at a dance. Another was conspicuously indisciplined and was sent to prison. A third keeps similar bad company and is locally expected to end up in the hands of the police. A fourth works on a farm but still lacks discipline. The girls have less lurid careers, though one was sent to a remand home. Several 'escaped' into very early marriage. The house in which another lived was condemned and pulled down while she was still at school.

We made no systematic follow-up of the pupils when they left school. The above details are of pupils who remained in the district and came to our notice. Naturally there would be a tendency for the more notorious or tragic cases to attract most attention, and we do know of a number of other deteriorators who settled down to jobs in the locality, and are socially co-operative. A few—but only a few—have in various ways done rather better than this. Several of the 'Improvers' are in universities and training colleges.

DETERIORATORS

Case No. 1

Jennifer was considered the most academically promising girl to pass through the junior school for many years; she worked hard and persevered over her difficulties. In the entrance examination for the grammar school she was one of the top five candidates. In her first year at the grammar school, however, her attainment in most subjects was poor. At the end of the first term she was demoted from the 'A' to the 'B' stream and further demoted to the 'C' stream as a result of the end-of-the-year examination. Her intelligence scores were not high, being only 105 on a Verbal group test and 112 on a Non-verbal. On the other hand other pupils with similar intelligence were reasonably successful in their studies; and Jennifer was reported by the junior school teachers to be conscientious and persevering.

The home was small and left little room for quiet study. Both parents were in unskilled employment but there were signs of poverty in the home. There were three other children in the family, Jennifer being the second born. There was no evidence of cultural pursuits; Jennifer herself bought paperback books and borrowed from the library. The home was very isolated and this girl of eleven had a long walk each day to an exposed bus stop before an hour's bus journey to school. The home seemed a happy one and the parents were encouraging, but they could not give Jennifer any help with her homework. Later her father was unable to work and Jennifer left school for a semi-skilled job and did not take the G.C.E. examination.

This was one of the most extreme of our cases but the deterioration in this instance could not be explained, as it could in so many cases, by lack of support or unhappiness in the home. Jennifer had no bad influences that we could detect. Her outside-school interests were painting, singing, needlework and reading. After careful study of the evidence we ascribed the deterioration to a combination of several factors. These were over-coaching at the junior school, lack of good ability (in spite of her high entrance position), lack of culture in the home and lack of adequate facilities for homework, and excessively long travel. Jennifer found the accumulation of difficulties too great for her and there was some falling off in application at the grammar school, her homework being of low standard.

Case No. 2

Jonathan also came in the first five out of over a hundred acceptances. He was reported to be a very steady worker, but rather shy. He was very good in English. At the grammar school he performed badly in English, Mathematics, Latin and the Modern Language, doing only fairly well in Woodwork, Art and General Knowledge. He was demoted to the 'B' stream at the end of the first term and to the 'C' stream at the end of the first year. His intelligence test scores were quite high—being 127 in a Verbal group test and 116 Non-verbal. His interests were philately, cycling and craft work. Jonathan, however, frequently played truant during his first year without his parents' knowledge. This frequent absence undoubtedly was a factor in his deterioration, but not the principal one. We discovered, unfortunately when it was too late, that the boy was born out of wedlock and he discovered this himself under circumstances which added to the shock and at a time which coincided with his entrance to the grammar school. This discovery had a considerable effect on his emotional outlook. He tended to avoid school and neglected his homework. He had slightly defective eyesight but did not wear spectacles during the first two years at the grammar school.

His home was adequate and comfortable and Jonathan had the use of his bedroom for indoor activities including homework. He was encouraged by his parents. His father was a skilled manual worker and there were two other children. His deterioration appeared to be a combination of emotional shock, truancy and his refusal to wear spectacles.

Case No. 3

Jeremy was placed just within the top quarter out of over a hundred acceptances. The junior school reported that he was 'a very active boy, good at Arithmetic, but his activities had to be directed and encouraged; he was easily distracted in the face of difficulties and sulked when his difficulties were ignored. He took an interest in all school activities, including games. He was near the top of his class'.

At the grammar school he performed badly in most subjects, only doing well in General Knowledge. As in the case of the previous pupils he was demoted to the 'B' stream at the end of the first term and to the 'C' stream at the end of the year. His intelligence level was not high, his Verbal score being 107 and the Non-verbal 104. In spite of his good marks in Arithmetic in the Entrance examination, Jeremy always showed a basic and consistent misunderstanding of operations involving multiplication by double figures—confusing the units and tens columns in the product. His progress in this type of subject in particular was hindered by his absenteeism. His conduct left much to be desired and his name frequently appeared in the punishment book. He had slightly defective eyesight but did not wear spectacles.

His mother was away from home, working, all day and his father was an unskilled shift worker. Jeremy very often had to cook for himself during the early evening and during the holidays. There were only two children. There was no poverty in the home, but the house was small and inadequate for study in the evening. It also lacked academic culture. Jeremy had some mechanical aptitude and spent many hours dismantling his father's motor-bike. Because of this and because the boy spent one-and-a-half hours in daily travel to and from school it was suggested to his parents that Jeremy could be transferred to a nearer technical school but the parents refused to co-operate.

Once again the sifting of the evidence showed that a number of factors were combining to cause Jeremy's deterioration in attainment. These were lack of strong support and lack of academic culture in the home, lack of persistence in face of difficulties, the refusal to wear spectacles, excessive travel, and finally absenteeism.

Case No. 4

Rosemary was just below the top third of 95 acceptances. The junior school reported that she was 'an extremely quiet and reserved child, who was very often seen quite alone. She had no great ability, but steadily and quietly persevered'. At the grammar school she did badly in Mathematics and General Science in particular; she had no strong subject. At the end of the year she was demoted to the lowest stream. Her Verbal intelligence score was not high (110) but other pupils of similar ability were successful in their work.

Rosemary lived in a mean street of small houses which con-sisted of two bedrooms, one sitting-room, one kitchen and a small auxiliary room; there were no modern conveniences. There were four beds to be shared between the parents and a very large number of children, of whom the eldest was in the late teens. The father was an unskilled labourer. The parents lacked pride of appearance and there were signs of squalor and lack of organisation in the home. The radio was constantly on and Rosemary had one in her own bedroom. She shared a bed with several other children and listened to the radio until about 9.0 p.m. No other child in the family had attended the grammar school. The parents wanted to 'give Rosemary her chance', but were quite unable to understand the part that they should play in doing this. The newspapers and journals taken by the family were the *Daily Herald, Daily Sketch, News of the World* and a comic. Rosemary did her homework directly after returning from afternoon school before the rest of the family settled down to a meal; but homework on a wet day was problematical in the extreme. The noise from the children in the house was continuous. Rosemary lacked encouragement in her work and was very reserved during the first year at the grammar school. We could find no reason for her deterioration other than the handicaps of her family background.

Case No. 5

David was placed about a third of the way down the Entrance list out of nearly a hundred acceptances. The junior school reported that he 'worked well at all times and was very keen about his work; he reached a good standard. All teachers spoke well of him. He was particularly good at Arithmetic problems'.

At the grammar school he did very badly in English (in which he was very weak in the Entrance examination), History, Latin, Algebra and Geometry; he did very well in Arithmetic and Woodwork. He was required to repeat the year's work. His deterioration cannot be ascribed to inferior ability as his Verbal Reasoning score was 122. His homework however, was often neglected.

David had a brother and a sister and they with their parents and an adult relative lived in a small house consisting of a kitchen, living-room and three bedrooms. The house lacked modern conveniences and was situated in a very mean street. David's father was in regular employment in a skilled occupation. During David's last year in the junior school the mother

73

neglected the home on two or three nights a week to attend social functions in the company of younger men. David took to stealing money (with another deteriorator). He was emotionally upset and though of good intelligence now deteriorated badly in his first year at the grammar school. There was a change in the family arrangements and his mother settled down, the family seeming reasonably happy, though there were some signs of financial struggle. David's progress at school became distinctly steadier.

David was rather young on entry and the repeating of the first year gave him time to find his feet and recover from his emotional upset. He even re-entered the 'A' stream during the third year, though he left school before sitting the G.C.E. examination. This case, however, was very exceptional, as very few pupils who were classed as deteriorators made any substantial recovery. The great majority remained at their low level of attainment and usually left school early.

Case No. 6

Priscilla was placed just below 30th position in the entrance examination out of 78 acceptances. The junior school reported that 'she was very quiet and reserved, but she always tried at her work and was keen to please; she responded well to a little encouragement'. Her rank order in class, however, was 'not very high'—whatever that rather ambiguous remark may mean.

In her first year at the grammar school she did badly in most subjects but did well in English and Latin. She did very little homework. She was demoted to the 'B' stream at the end of the first term and to the 'C' stream later. Her deterioration in attainment could not be ascribed to low ability as her group Verbal intelligence score was 125.

Our investigator found that the home was rather small, with some appearance of poverty. Her father was frequently out of work (he was a semi-skilled manual worker) and had not disciplined his indulgence in drink. He had left school before he was eleven years of age. The mother also lacked educational opportunity. She made few comments but the father ranged fluently from politics to education. He had taken much interest in Priscilla's homework before the Entrance examination but he found her work had got beyond him when she went to the grammar school.

Home discipline appeared rather slack; Priscilla attended the cinema regularly, twice a week on average. She was said to be happy at school and 'happy-go-lucky' in disposition. She was friendly with girls attending the secondary modern school as well as with grammar school girls. At home she had no quiet room in which to study. The only papers and journals taken in the home were *Daily Herald*, *The People*, *News of the World*, and the local weekly paper.

Priscilla did not recover from the lowest group ('C' stream). She sat the G.C.E. examination after five years at the grammar school and passed at the Ordinary Level in one subject out of six, namely Special Arithmetic.

Case No. 7

In the entrance examination Rachel came well above the half-way point in the order of merit though the junior school reported that 'she lacked initiative and ranked low in class order'. In the examination at the end of the first year she did badly in Foreign Languages and Mathematics except Arithmetic, but fairly well in English; she was in the bottom stream having been demoted from the upper half of the 'B' stream at the end of the first term. Her Intelligence results were good, her Non-verbal score being 123 and Verbal 121, so that her deterioration could not be ascribed to lack of general ability.

Rachel was a late arrival of a very large family. Her father, an unskilled manual worker, was vigorous though well over middle age. The mother had aged more than the father. The house was in a long ugly street of small houses and had three bedrooms, one sitting-room, one kitchen and a small wash-up. There were few books in the house. The family read the *Daily Herald*, *Mirror*, *Reynolds News* and *Sunday Dispatch*; also a local weekly paper. No children's papers were bought. There were signs of poverty although Rachel was clean and well dressed. Facilities for homework were very poor; there was lack of space and only one room had a fire.

The father was rather stern. He said he did not know his neighbours and did not mix in social events. (Rachel, however, seemed to be very fond of the Chapel and the Youth Club). Some of Rachel's sisters had attended the grammar school but her brothers had not been interested in education. Schools were not highly regarded by the parents and they were unenthusiastic about Rachel's performance at school.

Rachel had few close friends at the school and did not attend school parties and dances. She had little initiative and the Youth Club was her chief interest. Other interests were reading school library books, and the Band of Hope.

In her later career she remained in the bottom stream until she sat the G.C.E. (Ordinary Level) in eight subjects at the end of her five years at the school, passing in three. She sat again a year later and failed in all the subjects that she failed in at her first attempt.

Rachel clearly suffered from adverse home conditions, with poor facilities for homework. She also lacked initiative and persistence, this being aggravated by lack of encouragement by the parents.

Case No. 8

Edith was placed well above the half-way mark in the entrance examination in spite of the fact that the junior school reported that 'she could not be relied upon as to the amount of effort she would put into any piece of work. Her standard of work in any subject, therefore, varied considerably even from one day to another. She was placed low in rank order in the class'.

In her first year at the grammar school she deteriorated badly from her entrance position, obtaining very low marks in seven subjects. She had been demoted from the upper half of the 'B' stream to the 'C' stream at the end of the first term. Her ability was not high, her Non-verbal Intelligence Quotient being 102 and her Verbal Quotient 110. Her deterioration, however, seemed to be mainly due to lack of effort.

Her mother died when Edith was a baby and the father (semi-skilled) went away. Edith was brought up, lovingly, by the elderly grandparents on the father's side. The grandparents did not understand School Reports and thought that Edith was doing well! They thought that she worked so hard at school that she seldom had homework to do! What homework she did she was very impatient about and was much more interested in social activities in Church; she attended Youth Club and cinema once a week. There was evidently some poverty in the family and the buying of books would be luxury not to be indulged in: the family did not belong to a library. The house was small (two bedrooms, one sitting-room, one kitchen and an ante-room) and clean, though lacking indoor modern conveniences. Edith had not developed a hobby, nor was she interested in any cultural pursuit. The reading material was *Daily Mirror, The People, News of the World,* and the local weekly paper.

The grandparents had a high regard for both junior and grammar schools, but were incapable of fulfilling their role. There was lack of parental discipline and Edith formed outside friendships, mainly male, which aggravated the position.

Edith remained near the bottom of the lowest stream, left school before taking the G.C.E. examination, and married very early.

The home background was unfavourable. She had a weakness in Arithmetic, judging by the Arithmetic II entrance examination mark and by her Arithmetic Quotient (Schonell). This was the pupil, who at the end of the first year in the Grammar School, was discovered to be consistently multiplying wrongly by nought. Her Word Recognition score was also very low. She appeared to be more interested in social activities than in school work.

Case No. 9

Anne was about half-way down the order of merit list in the entrance examination. There was unfortunately no report on her from the junior school. During her first year at the grammar school she steadily deteriorated and obtained low marks in all subjects. At the end of the first term she was demoted from the upper half of the 'B' stream to the 'C' stream and remained there. Her conduct gradually became worse. Her Verbal Reasoning score was not obtained but her quotient in a Non-verbal test was 105 and in Figure Reasoning 111. Though these figures are not high, they would not in themselves explain her poor performance.

Anne had a very unhappy home. Her mother had left and her father, a semi-skilled manual worker, was working away from home. Anne lived with her grandfather who disliked her and showed it in his actions; the grandmother was more considerate. Anne often looked unkempt and neglected. She took to thieving of other children's property inside and outside school.

Though there was evidence to show that Anne found the work difficult in the 'B' stream, it is clear that the unhappy home background was the main cause of her deterioration. Her general conduct in the end necessitated exceptional treatment.

Case No. 10

Betty was placed very high in the entrance examination list. Her junior school reported that she was very promising academically, being hard-working and persevering. In order to attend the grammar school she had to meet an early bus some distance from her home and spent up to two hours travelling every day. During her first year she performed badly in most subjects but did fairly well in four. At the end of the first term she was demoted from the 'A' stream to the 'B' stream and at the end of the year went down to the 'C' stream. This rapid decline could not be ascribed wholly to lack of ability as her Verbal Reasoning Quotient was 111, her Non-verbal 115 and her Figure Reasoning 119.

Betty lived in a house which was too small for the family of six. It had no facilities for academic work. There were no standard books and no cultural pursuits. Betty bought cheap books of adventure, romance and school stories, and borrowed library books. The wages of her father, an unskilled labourer, were supplemented by the mother's unskilled work but there were signs of poverty in the home. The parents were sympathetic to Betty's efforts at school but they could not help her with academic work. She confessed to finding grammar school work difficult.

Betty did not sit for the G.C.E. examination and left to take up an unskilled job. The prospect of a maintenance grant could not alter her decision to leave. The unsupporting home background was the probable cause of her decline; the position was aggravated by long distance travel, and over-coaching at the junior school may have been responsible for her very high place in the entrance examination. This factor alone, however, could not be responsible for the dramatic change.

Case No. 11

John was placed well above the half-way level in the entrance examination list and had a reasonably good report from the junior school. He 'worked well, had initiative in tackling problems, but was untidy in setting out his work. He responded to encouragement. He was in the first ten in the Form'. He was placed—rather surprisingly—in the 'A' stream in the grammar school, but did rather badly and was therefore demoted to the 'B' stream. This demotion did not stop his deterioration and he was placed in the 'C' stream. He was absent for the Verbal Reasoning Test but his quotient for the Non-verbal was 106 and for Figure Reasoning .112. These quotients, though low, would scarcely explain his marked decline in attainment.

John's father was a semi-skilled manual worker. His family lived in a four-bedroom house, which also had a sitting-room, kitchen, bathroom and lavatory. It was an oldish building. Untidiness and lack of organisation generally characterised the home of this pupil. His mother spent her evenings convivially, outside her home, leaving the children to fend for themselves. John did the chores at home. His mother complained of lack of money (herself a heavy smoker) and declared that John should earn his living as soon as possible; John did his best by serving as an errand boy on Saturdays. The younger children were poorly dressed. John had no regular friends of his own age and he was an irregular member of the Boy Scouts. He became an artisan apprentice while in the lower school.

John's deterioration continued during his later short career at school. The main cause appeared clearly to be a deficient home background, with lack of encouragement by his parents. He was absent for 67 half-days during the first year, mainly in the second and third terms.

Case No. 12

This case study gives rise to a number of queries. Edward was placed comfortably in the top half of the order of merit in the entrance examination. However, the junior school reported, 'He spent two years in the upper class and sat the entrance examination to the grammar school twice. He was very slow with his work. It took him a long time to grasp any new rule and it required great patience on the part of the teacher. Rank order in Form—low'. In view of this report it is curious that Edward was placed in a fairly high position in the examination. Unless there was a slip the explanation would seem to lie in the fact that this was a second attempt. It would have seemed wise for the grammar school to have taken this into account and to have placed Edward in the 'C' stream rather than the 'B' stream. His Verbal Reasoning and Non-verbal Reasoning Quotients were only 100.

During his first year he did badly in most subjects and was demoted to the 'C' stream. After five years at school he took the G.C.E. examination but passed only in English.

Edward was the only child of elderly parents; his father, who was a skilled manual worker, had been ill for a long time. There was evidence of poverty in the home, and a cheerless atmosphere. The parents had no academic interests and did not understand their role in regard to the grammar school. The father studied the *Daily Herald* diligently; he was intolerant of opposing views (possibly a symptom of his physical condition). Home discipline was largely absent and the homework that Edward found difficult he did not attempt. The emotional tension in the home probably discouraged him from working as hard as he might have done, but there was some evidence to show that he found the work at 'B' level difficult. His persistence factor was not strong enough to enable him to overcome his difficulties.

Case No. 13

Richard was placed in the first quarter of the entrance examination list, having high scores in English and an astonishingly high one in the first Arithmetic paper. The report from the junior school was, however, not as promising. They reported,

'This boy had ability; but to get him to apply himself was one of the most difficult tasks. He was extremely highly-strung and needed more watching than the rest of the class put together. Concentration was often lacking and the degree of his effort varied considerably. He was between first and sixth in rank order in the Form'. At the grammar school he by no means lived up to the expectations aroused by his high entrance marks in English and Arithmetic and was demoted to the 'B' stream at the end of the first term. During the second term he contracted a complaint of the trachea (as a result of a chill) and was absent from school for six weeks. He lost ground academically and physically—and not only did he fail to recover from this unfortunate result of his absence but he rapidly deteriorated. This appeared to be due partly to an inherent weakness of a grammar school organisation—that there is no one in sufficiently close contact with cases like Richard's to understand the urgency of his need for help, and to provide special coaching. In the examination at the end of the year he did very badly indeed in English! and Arithmetic! and not very well in other subjects, though he did well in General Knowledge. As a result of the examination he was demoted to the 'C' stream.

In spite of his high mark in Arithmetic in the entrance examination he showed at the end of the first year in the Grammar School that he had no understanding of the basic processes of long division. He came from the same junior school as another deteriorator who showed the same weakness He had mislearnt parts of his multiplication tables.

Richard belonged to a small family, living in a small house, with two bedrooms and lacking modern conveniences. Both parents worked all day and returned just after six p.m., the father being in semi-skilled occupation and the mother in an unskilled job. The children lunched at school. His parents were very disappointed with Richard's academic progress; his mother, especially, stressed his pre-eminence in school examinations and sports when at the junior school; and (so she said) she could quote several names of failures at the grammar school, of boys and girls who were 'good scholars' at the junior school. According to the junior school Head teacher, Richard was outstanding at English and sports.

The lack of culture at Richard's home was unfortunate for him. The family did not lack money, but it was not spent on cultural pursuits, though the boys had plenty of story books. The *Daily Herald, Reynolds News* and the local weekly paper were the main family sources of news. The children attended Church on Sundays.

The chief cause of deterioration was the lack of a sufficiently steady persistence factor where academic work was concerned. The parents did not realise why the boy was deteriorating, could not help him academically, and did not realise how he might be helped in other ways. Though his deterioration had begun before his long absence, this missing of school work handicapped him still further. Grammar schools should be sufficiently well staffed to provide special help for such cases at least in subjects where later progress depends very much on the early foundation. His slight deafness was an additional handicap. The specific weakness in one of the basic processes of arithmetic could have affected his attitude to his work, but a persistent boy would have remedied this deficiency himself. He was, however, ill and absent from school for 63 half-days during the second term.

Case No. 14

Geoffrey came just above half-way in the order of merit in the entrance examination, doing much better in English than in Arithmetic. In the second Arithmetic paper he had a distinctly low mark and the junior school reported, 'This boy appeared very nervous when he commenced here (after transfer from another school). We found, however, that, given encouragement he could persevere, and a little interest in him reaped its reward. His rank was about half-way in the class.'

At the grammar school he was placed in the 'B' stream but had poor marks in most subjects except Science, Woodwork and Art, and was demoted to the 'C' stream at the end of the year. His deterioration could not be explained by his verbal reasoning ability as he had a quotient of 115. His Schonell Arithmetic Quotient was, however, very low. When examined diagnostically this test showed that Geoffrey consistently omitted 'internal' noughts in the quotients of division sums;

this was at the end of his first year at the grammar school. He did not recover from his position in the lowest stream and left school without sitting the G.C.E. examination. This family of three lived in a comparatively large house. His parents moved into this district from a neighbouring town and settled down happily; they took an active part in church activities. They had no financial worries. Geoffrey had made a great effort to 'pass' into the grammar school; he had slackened off after getting there and deteriorated—to his mother's disgust. She was inclined to 'nag' at him, whilst the father accepted the situation. Geoffrey was very fond of woodwork and was encouraged in his hobby. The parents suggested an engineering apprenticeship, which met with Geoffrey's approval.

Geoffrey's father had spent many years as a routine clerk. His parents considered education important but they themselves were not well educated. The family read *Daily Mirror, News of the World*, the local weekly paper, *Picture Post, John Bull* and *Illustrated*. Geoffrey did not lack adventure story books and encyclopaedic publications. He did not go to the cinema often. The impression was obtained that Geoffrey needed to regain confidence which his mother had lost for him. The relationship of the family to schools was lukewarm. Geoffrey had defective eyesight; he had been prescribed spectacles, but did not wear them. This could have affected not only his attainment but his attitude to school. His failure seemed to be due to a combination of factors, including some emotional difficulty at home and some innate lack of persistence.

Case No. 15

Roger was placed about mid-way in the order of merit in the entrance examination. His junior school reported, 'He needed constant encouragement to overcome his lack of initiative. He was slightly below middle in class position'. At the examination at the end of the first term in the grammar school he did badly and was demoted from the 'B' to the 'C' stream. He continued to do badly, however, except in English, Mathematics and two other subjects, so that at the end of the year he was placed in the 'D' stream. His Intelligence Quotient was 110 and that on a special test given later was 104. He left school early without sitting the G.C.E. examination, to be apprenticed.

While at the junior school Roger fell into the company of an older and less intelligent boy; as a result of pilfering, the juvenile court placed both on probation. Fortunately Roger withdrew his association with the older boy; the latter's further misdemeanours brought him more severe treatment.

Roger had a very unfortunate home background. The house was in a long street of small, ugly terraced houses. The mother seemed to lack geniality; she was frequently aggressive in her attitude towards the junior school, but she did not establish any relationship, aggressive or otherwise, with the grammar school. Roger was frequently scruffy in appearance and shabbily clothed. But the worst influence in the home was his father, an unskilled labourer, who probably made life intolerable for all members of the family. There would be little or no encouragement for Roger to progress at school with such a difficult father.

The home background was the overwhelming adversity in Roger's life. We can see no other cause for such drastic decline in his level of attainment.

Case No. 16

Michael's name appeared about a third of the way down the list of acceptances for the grammar school. His junior school reported 'He had the ability to do better; he lacked effort and persistence. His rank order in class was about half-way down the Form list'. When he went to the grammar school he gave in little or no homework and drifted steadily down the Form list. At the end of the first term he was sent down to the 'B' stream, and at the end of the year further demoted to the 'C' stream. His Verbal Intelligence Quotient was 108, which alone would not account for his poor attainment. He left school without sitting the G.C.E. examination and took a semi-skilled job.

The child relationship in Michael's home was simply chaotic. He had several brothers and sisters and there were several younger children of another marriage in the home. They all lived in a four-bedroom type house, one of the bedrooms being uninhabitable. Home conditions were like bedlam and the mother misruled with an iron hand. It is no wonder that Michael spent two evenings a week at a youth club and one (occasionally two) evening(s) at the cinema in his first year at the grammar school. There was little hope of improvement in the home conditions during Michael's school life. He was often absent from school for inadequate reasons. Both his father and step-father were semi-skilled workers. There was certainly some financial stringency and Michael received free meals at school.

Not surprisingly Michael made little effort. He lacked facilities for homework, lacked parental encouragement and had little to spare in ability (he tried the entrance examination twice). There was emotional upset in his home background.

IMPROVERS

Case No. 1

Mary's parents took her away from the local junior school because she was not making the progress that they wished, and placed her in a small private school. In the entrance examination she was placed comfortably above the half-way line, having done well in English and Essay. In the grammar school she was placed in the 'B' stream. In her first examination she came among the first ten in the Form in all literary subjects and was promoted to the 'A' stream. Her entrance I.Q. was 112 and later she obtained one of 117. After only four years at the grammar school she was allowed to sit the G.C.E. in five literary subjects and passed all of them with credit. Mary continued at school and gained an Advanced Level certificate with good grading in three languages.

Mary was an adopted child. Both 'parents' were ex-grammar school. Her 'mother' was formerly a clerk and her 'father' was a non-manual worker. Education was regarded with great respect and both 'parents' encouraged Mary with suitable reading books and provided her with good facilities for homework. Her 'mother' was apologetic in that she could only enjoy reading 'light' novels and women's journals; (there were two other young children in the family). Her 'father' read technical journals; both parents were members of a book club; they both shared the children's interests in Church, radio and television.

Mary was a quiet, rather reserved child. She was studious and had ability in Modern Languages, but seemed to have less ability in Arithmetic and Mathematics generally. She showed much persistence and single-mindedness in school work, and became established in the upper half of the 'A' stream. Her outside-school interests included reading, walking and Girl Guides, and she was very friendly with a girl from a private school. Undoubtedly she was aided in her improvement by the support and understanding she received at home.

Case No. 2

Margaret was placed in a very low position in the entrance examination. Her junior school reported, 'She was quiet, but persevered with her difficulties. Her work was neat, but on the whole she was slow in finishing it. She was not strong in health, and her performance at school work varied'. Because of her low position in the entrance examination Margaret was placed in the 'D' stream. However, she worked so commendably that she was promoted to the 'C' stream at the beginning of the second term and a later 'follow-up' showed her to be well established in the 'B' stream. Her Verbal Reasoning Quotient was certainly no higher than that of most of the deteriorators, being 109 on entrance and 103 on a different test later. In the G.C.E. examination which she sat five years after entrance, she gained passes in four literary subjects, Biology, General Science and Art. She then left school for vocational training in one of the professions.

Margaret seemed shy and a little nervous. She was anxious to perform well academically, and she took care with her work. She usually began her homework early, in a warm quiet room. Her mother was able to help her with Modern Language and even with Algebra and Geometry. But apart from this, there was little cultural background in the home, for books were not plentiful. The usual reading material was national newspapers—the *Daily Mail*, Sunday papers and women's journals. Although the father did not attend a grammar school, her parents were in favour of a grammar school education, at least as far as school certificate, but Margaret would be allowed to have a say in the length of school life. The impression was obtained that Margaret was well protected by elderly parents; the other daughter, several years older than Margaret, attended a secondary modern school.

All the evidence available indicated that Margaret possessed a high persistence factor. The home was encouraging to academic progress and sympathetic to the effort she made. She spent all her evenings on school work and seemed to have little time for her out-of-school activities.

Case No. 3

Stephen attended a small rural primary school and had a rather low place in the entrance examination. Unfortunately no report on his junior school activities is available. He was placed in the 'C' stream in the grammar school and in the end of the year examination he was in the first ten in the Form in four subjects and did well in all others. He was then promoted to the 'B' stream. His Verbal Reasoning Quotients were 109 on entrance and 116 on a different test later. After five years at the grammar school he sat for his G.C.E., Ordinary Level, and gained passes in six subjects. He then left school to enter a college of further education.

Stephen's parents considered a good education important and hoped that he would go to college or university on leaving the grammar school. His home was well supplied with books for his father's work—his father belonged to one of the professions—and suitable books for the children. His father had attended a grammar school, and although his mother lacked grammar school education, she did not lack culture. His parents indulged in social activities, and Stephen was able to share their interests; but since the home was rather isolated, there was little contact between him and other children in the neighbourhood (other than in organised meetings). Although there were no positive signs of poverty at the home, it was evident that Stephen would be obliged to shape a career. His parents encouraged him to enter fully into school life, including sports and games. He had a long bus journey to school.

There is evidence here for suggesting that a high persistence factor and a strong home background influence accounted for Stephen's academic progress. There was stability in the boy's character which appeared in reliability in his work within the limits of his ability.

Case No. 4

William came to the district only a few months before sitting the entrance examination and was also rather young. He was awarded a rather low position in the order of merit and was placed in the 'C' stream in the grammar school. Here he worked steadily and in the end of the year examination came in the first ten in six subjects including both English and Mathematics. He was therefore promoted to the 'B' stream. His Verbal Reasoning Ability Quotient was not particularly high; it was 112 on entrance and 110 by a later test. He took a very active part in school life generally and sat the Ordinary Level examination after five years, gaining eight passes. He later gained a good Advanced Level Certificate on the science side and left school for further education.

William had two changes of junior school in three years. He seemed to be weak in English as compared with Arithmetic. He was also rather slow in completing school work and not quick at oral work. His parents had attended a grammar school and were able to help William with his studies. His father belonged to the professional class and his mother did non-manual work before marriage. Conditions at home were very favourable to academic advancement, both in the way of books and conditions for homework. There was an assumption in the home that school life ends with Form Six but that education continues beyond that stage. Both of William's parents took a leading part in the social life of the neighbourhood and in cultural groups. The atmosphere in the home was academic and money was obviously being spent on books, journals and magazines. The radio was appreciated but had no nuisance value. William's out-of-school activities were centred on an outdoor life, namely camping, cycling, scouting.

William was below average age on entering the grammar school; a 'follow-up' two years later showed him well established in the upper-half of the 'B' stream, on performance in school examinations, which did not include age allowance. He possessed average persistence, and it is very probable that the home background was the strongest factor in his academic progress.

BIBLIOGRAPHY

AN effort has been made to increase the usefulness of this bibliography by making some differentiation between the value of the references *for the subject of the book*. Works of outstanding value are marked *. Works of importance are marked †, while the remainder represent research used for establishing points of lesser importance, official publications, and useful background reading.

ASSOCIATION OF EDUCATION COMMITTEES. *Early Leavers from Grammar Schools*. London, 1952.

†AULT, H. K., *An investigation into the causes of backwardness in Geography*. M.A. thesis, London, 1940.

†BIGGS, E. E., *An investigation into causes of backwardness in school mathematics*. M.A. thesis, London, 1951.

COLLINS, H., Premature Leaving from Grammar Schools. *Br. J. Educ. Psychol.*, Feb., 1955.

CROWTHER, G., Report *Fifteen to Eighteen*. Central Advisory Council for Education—England. H.M.S.O. London, Vol. 1, 1959, Vol. 2, 1960.

†DALE, R. R., *From School to University*. London, 1954.

†DALE, R. R., Review *Br. J. Educ. Studies*. 1957.

DEPARTMENT OF EDUCATION AND SCIENCE, Reports on Education, No. 17. London, Dec. 1964.

†DOUGLAS, J. W. B. *The Home and the School*. London, 1964.

*FLOUD, J. E.; HALSEY, A. H.; MARTIN, F. M. *Social Class and Educational Opportunity*. London, 1957.

*FRASER, E., *Home, Environment and the School*. Scottish Council for Research in Education, London, 1959.

*GLASS, D. V. (Edit.) *Social Mobility*. London, 1954.

†GREENALD, G. M., *An inquiry into the influence of sociological and physical factors on the trend of achievement in grammar school pupils*. Unpublished M.A. thesis, London, 1955.

HALSEY, A. H., GARDNER, L., Selection for Secondary Education. *Br. J. of Sociology*, March, 1953.

*JONES, C. V., *An enquiry into the causes of gross discrepancy between the performance of pupils in the 11 plus examination and their performance at the end of the first year in a Welsh grammar school.* M.A. thesis. Swansea, 1962.

†LEWIS, B. R. *Some relationships between comparative success and failure in Grammar Schools and certain aspects of personality.* M.A. thesis. London 1952.

MCINTOSH, D. M., *Promotion from Primary to Secondary Education* Scottish Council for Research in Education Publications, XXIX. London, 1948.

METCALFE, O., *The influence of socio-economic factors on school progress and personality development.* M.A. thesis, Birmingham, 1950.

MINISTRY OF EDUCATION, *Fifteen to Eighteen.* Central Advisory Council for Education—England, H.M.S.O. Vol. 1, 1959; Vol. 2, 1960. (Crowther Report).

*Early Leaving Central Advisory Council for Education, H.M.S.O., 1954.

Half Our Future Central Advisory Council for Education, London, 1963. (Newsom Report).

THE NATIONAL FOUNDATION FOR EDUCATIONAL RESEARCH, LONDON. *Allocation Study,* No. 5 (1955).

†OSMEND, E. L. J., *Some problems of selection for secondary grammar schools with special reference to misfits.* M.A. thesis, Birmingham, 1951.

RICHARDSON, S. C. *The use of attainment tests. Jnl. of Inst. Educ.,* Durham, Sept. 1956

*RUSHTON, J., *The relation between personality assessment and some measures of mental capacity used in secondary school selection.* Unpublished M.Ed. thesis, University of Manchester, 1963.

SANDON, F., *The comparative effect on progress of (a) many short, and (b) one long absence in a secondary grammar school. Br. J. Educ. Psychol.* June, 1938.

†SCHONELL, F. J., *Causes of backwardness.* Year Book of Education, London, 1936.

The Psychology and Teaching of Reading. London, 1946, 2nd ed.

Diagnosis of Individual difficulties in Arithmetic. London, 1949, reprint.

STOTT, D. H. *Unsettled Children and their Families.* London, 1956.

VALENTINE, C. W., *The Reliability of Examinations*. London, 1932.
*VERNON, P. E., (Edit.) *Secondary School Selection*. London, 1957.
*WHALLEY, G. E. *The effect of social class on the academic progress of boys within a boys' grammar school*. M.Ed. thesis. Durham, 1961.

INDEX

Ability, *see* Aptitude *and* Intelligence
Absence, 13, 35–6, 71–2, 79, 85
Academic aptitude, *see* Aptitude
Academic deterioration, *see* Deteriorators *and* Deterioration
Academic progress,
  factors affecting, *see* Deterioration
  influence of home background, *see* Home influence
  size of family, 19–21, 24
Academic improvement, *see* Improvers
Age, school leaving, 25, 29
Aptitude, 8–13, 41, 51–3
Arithmetic,
  absence from school, 13
  deteriorators, 71, 77, 81, 82–3
  emotional factors, 13
  factors affecting progress, 52
  standardised, 7
A.E.C., 24
Attainment, *see* Deteriorators, Improvers, Home influence etc.
Attainment tests, *see* Tests
AULK, H. K., 24

Bias, danger, 69
BIGGS, E. E., 13
BOOTLE, 23, 64
Border-line cases, 10
BRITISH PSYCHOLOGICAL SOCIETY, 8
Buildings, 40, 61

Case studies, 44, 68–88
'Ceiling effect', 10–11, 21
Cinema, 25, 75, 77
Class size, 61
COLLINS, H., 25

Comprehensive school, 67
Criteria,
  see Deteriorators
  see Improvers
Culture conflict, 66
Cultural level, of the home, *see* Home influence
Curriculum, 61

DALE, R. R., 1, 25
Delinquency, 19, 78, 84
Demotion,
  criterion, 4
  procedure, 4
DEPARTMENT OF EDUCATION AND SCIENCE, 30; *see also* MINISTRY
Deteriorators,
  ability, 9–11, 73, 75, 81, 82
  arithmetic, 13, 52, 71, 77, 81–3
  attainment, sex differences, 32, 40–3, 45, 48–9
  attitude to work, 51, 53–4, 67
  case studies, *see* Chapter VII
  control groups, 8–9, 12, 16–21
  definition, 3–4, 7
  disharmony in the home, 26–8, 54–5, 58
  emotional factors in arithmetic, 13
  emotional instability, 12, 54, 78
  health gradings, 34
  homework facilities, *see* Home influence
  I.Q. range, 9, 52
  lack of parental support, 24–6
  later careers, 3, 69
  minor ailments, *see* Health
  number of, 3
  out-of-school friends, 37, 68, 75, 77

Deteriorators—*cont.*
 out-of-school interests, 25, 68
 parental education, 16–18, 48,
  55–6
 premature leaving, *see* Premature
  leaving
 rank order 11+ entrance, 10–11
 sex difference, *see* Deteriorators,
  attainment
 social class, 14–16, 24, 55–9
 standard of work, 4, 12–13, 52
 subject preference, 5, 37–8
 word recognition quotient, 12–13
Deterioration, causes,
 absence, 35–6
 attitude of parents, 17, 24–6, 57–8
 attitude to school subjects, 37–8,
  53–4
 emotional, 13, 54, 58
 family size, *see* Family size
 games, 33
 health, 33–5; *see also* Health,
  minor ailments
 inherited personal characteristics,
  59
 intelligence, lack of, 9–10, 44–6,
  51, 59
 overcoaching, 37, 42–3, 70, 79
 persistence, lack of, 32–3, 44, 72,
  76, 80, 82, 83
 poverty, 23–4, 56, 77
 principal factors, 44–7
 social class, 14, 55–9
 standard of education of parents,
  see Parental education
 transition from primary to secondary school, 37, 60
Discipline, *see* Home influence
DOUGLAS, J. W. B., 17, 41

'Early Leaving', MINISTRY REPORT,
 16, 22, 26
Education, parental, *see* Parental
 education
Educational guidance,
 Tutor, 63–4
 Officer, 64

Emotional,
 disturbance, 13, 14, 44–5, 54–8,
  71, 74
 in arithmetic testing, 13
 in the home, 26–8, 80, 83–4
 in word recognition testing, 12
Entry, grammar school, 4, 40
 percentage of age group, 40
 see Examination
English, standardised test, 7
Estimates, teachers, 10
Examination, entrance, 7, 11, 40–1,
 50
Extra-mural coaching, 37
Eye-sight, *see* Health, minor ailments

Failures, *see* Deteriorators
Family size, 18–21, 68, 78
 delinquency, 19
 deteriorators, 19–21, 24, 57, 72,
  75, 78, 84
 improvers, 20–1
 poverty and, 19, 24, 56–7
 social class and, 19–21
First born, 20, 48, 57
FLOUD, J. E. *et al.*, 19, 26 40
Form teachers, *see* Teachers
FRASER, E., 18, 24, 27

Games, 33
GARDNER, L., 60
GLASS, D. V., 6, 46
Grammar School, The, 1–2, 36–7
 background, 5
 character, 5–6
 entry, 5
 entry from School X, 40–1
 reforms, 61–7
Grant, maintenance, 23–4, 78
GREENALD, G. M., 18, 20
Guidance, educational, *see* Educational guidance

HALSEY, A. H., 60
Health, 13, 33–5
 minor ailments, 35, 71, 82, 83
Hertfordshire, South-west, 26

Index

For Product Safety Concerns and Information please contact our EU
representative GPSR@taylorandfrancis.com
Taylor & Francis Verlag GmbH, Kaufingerstraße 24, 80331 München, Germany

www.ingramcontent.com/pod-product-compliance
Lightning Source LLC
Chambersburg PA
CBHW050719280326
41926CB00088B/3285

9 7 8 0 4 1 5 8 6 3 9 6 4